Sensory Issues and High-Functioning Autism Spectrum and Related Disorders

Sensory Issues and High-Functioning Autism Spectrum and Related Disorders:

Practical Solutions for Making Sense of the World

Second Edition

Brenda Smith Myles, PhD, Kelly Mahler, MS, OTR/L, and Lisa A. Robbins, PhD

Illustrated by Penny Chiles

Foreword by Winnie Dunn, PhD, and Judy Endow, MSW

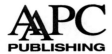

©2014 AAPC Publishing
P.O. Box 23173
Shawnee Mission, Kansas 66283-0173
www.aapcpublishing.net

Publisher's Cataloging-in-Publication

Myles, Brenda Smith.

Sensory issues and high-functioning autism spectrum and related disorders : practical solutions for making sense of the world / Brenda Smith Myles, Kelly Mahler, and Lisa A. Robbins ; illustrated by Penny Chiles ; foreword by Winnie Dunn, and Judy Endow. -- Second edition. -- Shawnee Mission, Kansas : AAPC Publishing, c2014.

p. ; cm.
ISBN: 978-1-937473-77-8
LCCN: 2014941554
    Revised edition of: Asperger syndrome and sensory issues : practical solutions for making sense of the world / Brenda Smith Myles ... [et al.]. Shawnee Mission, Kan. : Autism Asperger Pub. Co., c2000.
    Includes bibliographical references and index.
    Summary: This book explains how many children with high-functioning ASD relate to the world through their senses. The book reviews sensory integration terminology and a discussion of how the sensory systems impact behavior. It also takes an in-depth look at sensory issues associated with ASD. Assessment tools can assist children in pinpointing sensory characteristics. Intervention strategies and case studies are also outlined.--Publisher.

    1. Autism spectrum disorders in children--Treatment. 2. Autism spectrum disorders--Treament. 3. Autism spectrum disorders--Patients--Rehabilitation. 4. Asperger's syndrome in children--Treatment. 5. Asperger's syndrome--Treatment. 6. Autism in children--Treatment. 7. Sensory integration dysfunction in children--Treatment. 8. Sensory integration dysfunction--Treatment. 9. Sensorimotor integration-- Handbooks, manuals, etc. I. Mahler, Kelly J. II. Robbins, Lisa A. III. Chiles, Penny. IV. Title.

RJ506.A9 M975 2014
618.92/85882--dc23   1406

This book is dedicated

to the children, parents,

and educators who have

been our teachers.

FOREWORD TO FIRST EDITION

Imagine all the ways that we might describe the experiences of living across a span of 70 years. In some ways, perspectives become more complex as we become increasingly aware of more and more aspects of living. But in other ways, across this length of time, the simplicity and rhythm of living become more apparent. In addition, both of these ways of characterizing living would be different from the way in which we would have characterized each of the decades within the 70 years, because the accumulation of knowledge and insight informs us in a unique way from any other single experience. When we can move forward and backward in our thinking about phenomena, patterns can emerge that were not evident in our actual experience of them as individual parts.

We are experiencing this same 70-year perspective when examining and addressing the issues of high-functioning autism spectrum disorder (HF-ASD). In 1944 Hans Asperger provided an initial description of a group of children who were unique from any others he had encountered. In the 70 years since then, professionals have increasingly recognized the uniqueness and complexity of this disorder once referred to as Asperger Syndrome and now HF-ASD. Although many of the core behaviors that contribute to the diagnosis of HF-ASD have remained surprisingly constant, professionals have continued to search for underlying factors that might be present to yield these core behaviors. Professionals have believed that by understanding underlying factors we have more precise options for effective intervention to support successful and satisfying lives for persons with HF-ASD and their families.

I don't think it is any coincidence that, during the "Decade of the Brain," professionals began to interpret some of the core behaviors of HF-ASD as indicative of difficulties with sensory processing. This was a period in our culture that was focused on neuroscience to explain many human phenomena. For example, from a sensory processing point of view, core behaviors such as "difficulty discerning relevant from irrelevant stimuli" might indicate an inability to screen incoming sensory information properly for use in daily life. And now, finally, due to many of the advancements during the "Decade of the Brain," sensory processing issues have been formally recognized as a core underlying factor of HF-ASD and have been included as a diagnostic criterion in the recent release of the *Diagnostic and Statistical Manual of Mental Disorders, 5th Revision* (American Psychiatric Association, 2013).

In order to continue advancing our knowledge, we will have to further study the impact of these sensory processing challenges. We have to create systematic methods for applying a sensory processing perspective to the daily life challenges of persons with HF-ASD and measure the effectiveness of these methods. Families and persons with HF-ASD must understand the challenges in their own terms so that they can be informed participants and provide insights about their own lived experiences. Family and persons with HF-ASD provide the 70-year perspective, because they can reflect forward and backward as they consider the ideas of sensory processing, and give us insights we cannot gain from merely observing.

This book contributes to knowledge development by providing friendly explanations about complex phenomena. This approach invites families to participate in the perspective taking, so they can share both the complexity and the rhythms of living that come along with the experience of HF-ASD with those of us who are merely observers (i.e., the professionals). Only with all the perspectives can we hope to expose the truth.

Winnie Dunn, Ph.D., OTR, FAOTA

Winnie Dunn, PhD, OTR, FAOTA, is professor and chair of the Department of Occupational Therapy Education at the University of Kansas. She has written many books and articles on service provision in schools and on sensory processing in daily life. In 1999, her research on sensory processing with children culminated in the publication of the Sensory Profile, a caregiver reporting measure of children's responses to sensory events in daily life. She continues this work with infants, toddlers, adults and older adults, currently collecting standardization and validation data nationwide. Most recently, she has authored or coauthored two books about best practices: Best Practice Occupational Therapy in Community Settings with Children and Families *and* Measuring Occupational Performance: A Guide to Best Practice Assessment, *both published by SLACK.*

Dr. Dunn has received many honors throughout her career. She was named Fellow of the American Occupational Therapy Association (FAOTA) and received the Award of Merit for significant contributions to the profession. She was named to the Academy of Research of the American Occupational Therapy Foundation, and has received research awards from her university as well. In the spring of 2000, she was named the Eleanor Clark Slagle Lecturer for 2001, the highest honor given in the profession, for her significant contributions to knowledge development.

FOREWORD TO SECOND EDITION

Today we know that sensory differences affect most individuals with autism spectrum disorder (ASD), as evidenced by the research outlined in this book. Yet, there remains a big gap between this knowledge and the practical implementation of effective sensory supports for all of our students needing them.

In my consultation with schools, agencies, and families on behalf of those with ASD, I have come across numerous examples of this gap. *Sensory Issues and High-Functioning Autism Spectrum and Related Disorders* fills this gap, thus meeting the needs of parents, care providers, teachers, and school staff as they strive to care for, teach, and meet the needs of individuals across the day.

In the spirit of practicality, let me outline the kinds of gaps between knowledge and practice I see along with how this book fills those gaps.

- *The gap in understanding sensory implications for behavior*

  We all look at the world from our own place of understanding. We assign meaning to behavior we see according to what that behavior would mean if we were engaged in it. Most of the time, this innate strategy of assigning meaning to behavior we see in others works well, so we keep using it. However, when the individual engaged in behavior that isn't working well for those around him has sensory system differences, the meaning assigned to his behavior may not be accurate. This is important because our interventions are based on the meaning we assign to behavior. Therefore, when the meaning is incorrect, the interventions are unsuccessful.

  With *Sensory Issues and High-Functioning Autism Spectrum and Related Disorders*, we don't have to continue haphazardly guessing why anyone is behaving in an unconventional manner when there is a sensory basis for the behavior. Instead, we can read about how sensory processing differences in the brain lead to behaviors in those we love, care for, and teach. A practically concise review of the important work of Winnie Dunn gives the reader an understanding of the basis to the often-heard sentiment …"if only I knew why he was doing that."

  If this is your gap, read Chapter 1, which discusses four types of common sensory issues often experienced by individuals with ASD (overresponsivity, underresponsivity, craving, and discrimination difficulty). These are the sensory answers to the question, "Why does he do that?"

  If your gap is "How do I know if the behavior is sensory related?," read Chapter 2. Each of eight sensory systems functions and their role in our body is explained and interfaced with the four types of common sensory issues. In addition, an easy-to-use chart lists commonly observed behaviors along with possible sensory reasons for the behavior for each of the eight senses.

- *The gap in assessing sensory processing issues*

  For those tasked with conducting a more formal sensory assessment, the gap may lie in knowing what sorts of assessment tools are available today and how to use them. If so, Chapter 3 is for you! It includes a table of 10 sensory assessment tools used today along with specific information on each, allowing you to easily compare and contrast and to see at a glance what tools apply to which individuals. Additionally, 10 techniques for evaluating those with ASD along with guidelines for observations will help fill in this gap area.

- *The gap in implementing sensory interventions*

  If your gap involves the question "What are the best sensory interventions for this particular individual?," you will find your answers in Chapter 4, where evidence-based practices and sensory interventions are discussed along with relevant research. Also, a practical outline and description of 20 top resources – programs and publications specifically addressing various sensory regulation needs of those with ASD – will enable you get a quick understanding of what is available that has been shown to work.

  If your gap involves the question "What should I try?" or "Where do I start?," you will love looking over the 18-page table that outlines kinds of behavior, their sensory interpretations, and specific practical classroom intervention ideas.

- *The gap in supporting sensory needs of individuals across the day*

  And finally, if your gap involves how to put together a comprehensive program that makes practical sense over the course of the day in a way that can be easily implemented, Chapter 5 is for you. Four models that do just this are presented to help you decide when to use which models with which individuals. This includes comprehensive models for use in school, in the community, and interpersonally (addressing friendship) to match the needs of those with ASD.

This is the most comprehensively practical sensory-related book I have read to date! I will be carrying this book along as I go on consultations because it addresses most of the gaps I see between knowing sensory issues are important for individuals with ASD and related disorders and understanding how to meet them in a way that supports those of us on the autism spectrum to be all we can and all we want to be as we grow up and take our place in this world.

Judy Endow, MSW, autism consultant; http://www.judyendow.com

TABLE OF CONTENTS

INTRODUCTION

Parents typically "know" the unique characteristics of their children and are often able to anticipate their own child's actions based on what they know about children in general. But some children present challenges that make it difficult for both teachers and parents to anticipate how they may react to certain situations. Their behaviors may seem puzzling, mysterious, even frightening.

On her blog, The AWEnesty of Autism (http://www.awenestyofautism.com), Kathy Hooven shared the following experience she had with her son, Ryan.

> Before my brain knew, before the doctor actually said the words, "Your son has an autism spectrum disorder," my heart knew, but between my son's wailing and my own inner voice chanting, "Please, don't let it be autism, please don't let it be autism," my brain could not hear my terrified heart. It took a soccer referee's whistle to finally break through my soundproof brain and allow me listen to my heart.
>
> On a brisk fall day, while at his brother's soccer game, my three-year-old son was literally burrowing his head into my chest trying to escape the bright sun, the wind, and the unforgiving, unexpected screech of the referee's whistle. With cries of "no, no, no" screamed in my ear as my son's rubber sneakers pinched and bruised the flesh on my thighs and with his head trying to push its way into my heart so I could finally hear him, my son was trying to tell me that the sun, the wind, and the whistle were just too much for him. My poor boy's sensory system was being taxed in a way that I didn't understand. But as I gazed at all the other children laughing and playing in the bright sun, unaffected by the cold wind whipping through their hair and showing not even the tiniest flinch at the shrill, piercing whistle, I knew my son was different. I knew it was time to block out my frightened inner voice and to finally listen to my heart. (Used with permission.)

Just as Ryan demonstrated puzzling reactions to seemingly typical sensations, so do many other children. You may recognize some of these reactions in Figure I.1 as being typical of some of the children you know. Some children experience several of these challenges whereas others may experience one or two. Some behaviors and reactions are problematic and interfere with work or play, others do not compromise the success of these interactions. What is the difference and how can we reduce or eliminate the occurrence of the frustrations experienced by individuals with sensory differences?

Whether the child demonstrates one or a multitude of perplexing behaviors, finding an explanation helps you not only to make sense of what is occurring but also to anticipate similar reactions in the future.

This book will cover puzzling behaviors that may have a sensory base. In particular, we will look at behaviors exhibited by individuals with high-functioning autism spectrum disorders (HF-ASD), including those with the previous DSM-IV diagnosis of Asperger Syndrome.

Until recently, sensory issues were often overlooked as a root cause of the difficulties experienced by individuals with HF-ASD, mainly because we only had anecdotal information. Numerous people with HF-ASD shared with the world what it was like to live with these sensory issues and the challenges they presented. But despite how powerful these personal accounts were, they were not enough to convince everyone of the significant impact of sensory issues.

Often this oversight resulted in greater frustrations because no matter how well intended and well designed, many interventions did not address the actual root of the difficulties. Furthermore, many times this lack of widespread acceptance of the impact of sensory issues resulted in people being "forced" to endure situations and environments that were highly uncomfortable and distressing to them.

We now finally have research and literature that support the subjective information. Sensory difficulties were even recently added as a diagnostic criterion in the *Diagnostic and Statistical Manual of Mental Disorders, 5th Edition* (American Psychiatric Association [APA], 2013). Hopefully, now sensory issues will receive the focus and consideration they deserve, and the information presented in this book will help make that process as seamless and easy as possible.

Chapter 1 presents an overview of sensory-related terminology, including descriptions of effective and ineffective sensory processing. Chapter 2 takes an in-depth look at the common sensory issues associated with HF-ASD. Chapter 3 covers both formal and informal assessment tools that can assist in pinpointing sensory characteristics. Chapter 4 offers a series of intervention strategies that can be used in supporting common sensory difficulties. Finally, Chapter 5 presents methods for proactively embedding sensory supports across the day and in a variety of environments.

Throughout these chapters, the reader will learn about the Sensory Gang, a busy, hard-working squad compromised of members representing each sensory system. With the help of the Sensory Gang, the book will attempt to explain each sense and how many children with HF-ASD relate to the world through their senses.

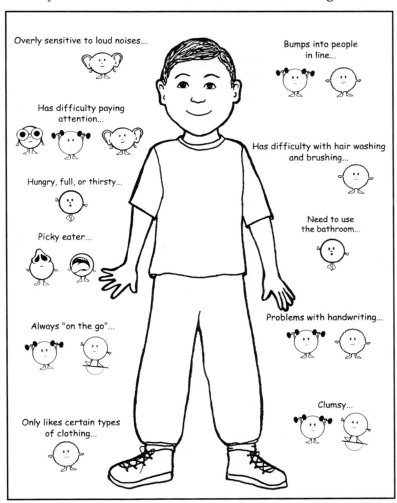

Figure I.1. Sample of sensory characteristics of the typical child with HF-ASD.

THE SENSORY GANG

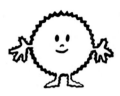

Ms. Tactile

People say I am so touchy-feely! I can't help it! From head to toe and all over, my skin keeps me "in touch" with the world. Even inside my mouth I feel things – light touch, deep pressure, hard or soft, sharp or dull, vibration, temperature and ohhhhh … the pain!

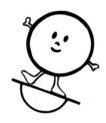

Mr. Vestibular

I keep everything "right with the world"! Because of me, you can deal with gravity when you are moving, no matter the direction or speed. Even when standing or sitting still, I am very important because of my sense of balance. Posture and muscle tone depend on the signals I interpret from the inner ear.

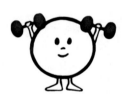

Ms. Proprioception

I do more than just push and pull, flex and stretch, pry and press! Information coming from my joints, muscles and tendons helps me adjust my body position for smooth movements with just the "right amount" of pressure. People say I am important for good "motor planning" when this information is accurate.

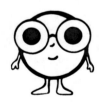

Ms. Visual

I've got my eyes on you! I am on the lookout to deliver valuable details about what I see. Color, contrast, line, shape, form and movement have a part in how you perceive the world. My messages (with the collaboration of my friends) help determine what to pay attention to and what to ignore as well as help direct your actions and movements.

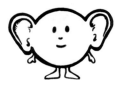

Ms. Auditory

Do you hear what I hear? I don't mean to whine, but I can get your attention, too. Listen to me, please, I'm all ears. It's not just about volume – consider also tone, pitch, rhythm and sequence of sounds. Processing me can be difficult, but it is necessary if I am to be understood. If I don't have the others help out, I'm just noise … sigh.

Mr. Gustatory

Ah, to savor the "sweet taste of success," or was it bitter or salty? Maybe sour or spicy? Taste buds and saliva are the grounds for my great sensory contributions. I often get no respect but one thing's for sure, I know "what I like!" By the way, I am intricately linked with Ms. Olfactory.

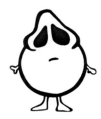

Ms. Olfactory

Although some consider me not as refined as my other sensory friends, I go way back in time – kind of a survival thing. Strong memories are associated with certain smells. I subjectively consider the odor, especially when Mr. Gustatory is around. Remember, the "nose knows" and … "Don't forget to stop and smell the roses."

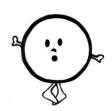

Mr. Interoception

Did you feel that? I am responsible for helping you notice the inside of your body. I let you know important things like when you are hungry, full, or thirsty, or when you need to use the bathroom. Pay attention to me … I'll also send you clues about your emotions. Fast heartbeat and upset stomach could mean that you are feeling anxious. Calm breathing often signals that you are relaxed and content.

CHAPTER 1

Sensory Processing

Sensory processing can be quite technical and is sometimes an intimidating topic to tackle. However, since sensory issues can have a profound impact on a person's well-being and general functioning, it is imperative to expand our understanding in this area. It is our hope that sensory processing becomes common knowledge not only for those directly impacted by HF-ASD, but for the entire public. Ideally, improved understanding of sensory issues will allow for a more sensory-friendly world.

Before diving into the topic of sensory processing, there are a few important points to note.

1. **Sensory processing.** Our nervous system is responsible for the very important job of "making sense" of the sensory world. Basically, sensory information goes in and behavior comes out. Exactly how that link occurs and the words chosen to describe the process may be expressed in different ways by individuals or groups of individuals attempting to identify and explain behavior from a sensory perspective (Kwakye, Foss-Feig, Cascio, Stone, & Wallace, 2011). In other words, a neuroscientist uses words that refer to a specific neurophysiological action whereas an occupational therapist may use the same or similar term in a more global, behavioral manner. As the theory of sensory processing continues to evolve and the scientific community learns more about how the nervous system works, additional terminology is likely to emerge.

2. **Recent changes in the field of sensory processing.** The last decade has seen significant contributions to our knowledge about the sensory systems. These recent advancements have enhanced not only our understanding about but also our ability to support sensory processing difficulties in individuals with HF-ASD. Along with these changes, adaptations to classification and terminology have occurred. For the sake of

this book, and for gaining the best understanding of the sensory issues that individuals with HF-ASD may face, in the following we have combined the most common thinking regarding sensory processing.

3. **Sensory Processing Disorder (SPD).** SPD and HF-ASD are not one and the same! They are separate diagnoses. A child can have SPD and not have HF-ASD. Conversely, a child can have HF-ASD and not have SPD. However, because the latter is much less likely to happen – rates of SPD among individuals with HF-ASD may be as high as 95% (Baker, Lane, Angley, & Young, 2008; Baranek et al., 2006; Dunn, Myles & Orr, 2002; Tomchek & Dunn, 2007) – it is of utmost importance to understand current thinking about SPD. Hopefully, with a solid understanding of sensory processing and SPD, we will be able to make "sense" of the way individuals with HF-ASD view and experience the world and, as a result, support them when needed.

Learning About the Eight Senses – The Sensory Gang

Eight senses? Yep! Most of us are familiar with the five most talked-about members of the Sensory Gang: Visual (sight), Auditory (sound), Tactile (touch), Gustatory (taste), and Olfactory (smell). But there are also three less known senses: Vestibular (balance or head position in relation to gravity), Proprioception (body awareness or input from joints and muscles) and Interoception (awareness of how our internal organs feel). In order to think about each sense, let's take a detailed look at the seemingly easy task of getting on the school bus.

As you climb the bus steps, you are able to do so without looking down at your feet (proprioception). Once you have entered the bus, you quickly scan all the seats, looking for an empty spot (visual). You find an empty seat but suddenly hear a friend calling your name from the back of the bus (auditory). You see him wave you back to sit with him (visual), so you swiftly move toward the back. On your way down the aisle, your foot brushes against a bag another student has left in the middle of the floor (tactile). Without even looking down, you jump over the bag and land safely in your seat next to your friend (proprioception).

With everybody now on board, the bus starts up and lurches forward on its way to the next stop. You adjust your body so that it remains upright on the seat (vestibular). The bus is loud, but you are able to listen to the story that your friend has started telling you (auditory). As you are answering a question your friend asks, you simultaneously smell chocolate (olfactory) and begin searching for the source (visual). You spot the culprit – a friend sitting nearby eating a candy bar. Your stomach starts to growl, and you realize that you forgot to eat breakfast (interoception). You ask your friend to share a piece of the candy, but before he can pass it to you, a car horn blares outside (auditory). While you are glancing out the window (visual), you reach behind you and grab the chocolate (proprioception). The chocolate is a little warm and mushy (tactile), but you don't care. You pop it in your mouth and enjoy the sweetness (gustatory) as you resume your conversation with your friend.

Whew!! All of this has happened in about 90 seconds, and the most exhausting part is that your senses did a lot more work than we had space to mention!

Clearly, the Sensory Gang has an important job to do. They are constantly collecting and taking in valuable sensory information about ourselves as well as the surrounding environment. As early as into 10 weeks of development, the fetus has a few developed senses that can take in sensory information. This incoming information may contribute to the developing brain and central nervous system. As the fetus grows in utero, so do the sensory systems. This is why so many parents play classical music or read aloud during pregnancy to stimulate growth and development of the fetus.

Each sensory system has receptors or specialized cells throughout the body that take in information about the world. The information gathered by these sensory receptors becomes the starting points for delivering messages to the brain and the rest of the central nervous system. Some parts of the body have an increased density or higher number of receptors compared to other parts of the body. For example, your mouth and hands have more receptors in the same amount of body surface than your back or leg, providing more sensory messages for processing. Table 1.1 provides detailed information about the receptor location and the function of each of the eight sensory systems.

Table 1.1
Location and Functions of the Sensory Systems

System	Location	Function
Tactile (touch)	**Skin** – density of cell distribution varies throughout the body. Areas of greatest density include mouth, hands, and genitals.	Provides information about the environment and object qualities (touch, pressure, texture, hard, soft, sharp, dull, heat, cold, pain).
Vestibular (balance)	**Inner ear** – stimulated by head movements and input from other senses, especially visual.	Provides information about where our body is in space, and whether or not we or our surroundings are moving. Tells about speed and direction of movement.
Proprioception (body awareness)	**Muscles and joints** – activated by muscle contractions and movement.	Provides information about where a certain body part is and how it is moving.
Visual (sight)	**Retina of the eye** – stimulated by light.	Provides information about objects and persons. Helps us define boundaries as we move through time and space.
Auditory (hearing)	**Inner ear** – stimulated by air/sound waves.	Provides information about sounds in the environment (loud, soft, high, low, near, far).
Gustatory (taste)	**Chemical receptors in the tongue** – closely entwined with the olfactory (smell) system.	Provides information about different types of taste (sweet, sour, bitter, salty, spicy).
Olfactory (smell)	**Chemical receptors in the nasal structure** – closely associated with the gustatory system.	Provides information about different types of smell (musty, acrid, putrid, flowery, pungent).
Interoception (inside body)	**Inside of your body** – helps the body "feel" the internal state or conditions of the body.	Provides information such as pain, body temperature, itch, sexual arousal, hunger and thirst. It also helps bring in information regarding heart and breathing rates and when we need to use the bathroom.

An Overview of Sensory Processing

As mentioned, the receptors for each sensory system are constantly taking in information from the environment and from our bodies and sending it to our brain. The brain, in turn, tries to organize and make sense of all this information and produce a response. This is called sensory processing.

In other words, sensory processing refers to the way the brain and the nervous system receive sensory messages and turn them into responses (Miller, 2006). For example, when you step on a sharp pin, your tactile (touch) sense sends a message to your brain; your brain translates the message (pain/danger!!) and immediately sends a message to your foot (PULL BACK!). This process occurs automatically and instantaneously. You don't need to think about it.

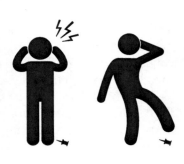

Here's another way to look at sensory processing. If we compare our bodies to a computer, our brain would be the central processing unit (CPU) that detects, regulates, interprets, and sends messages to the rest of the body. The CPU (aka brain) sends messages that help us to regard, disregard, seek out or avoid sensation. This, in turn, maintains or increases our feelings such as comfort, excitement and rest, and enables us to have positive interactions with objects and peers.

Conversely, the CPU (aka brain) also influences how we try to avoid sensory input that is painful, uncomfortable or stressful. Whether it's cold outside, we have a stomachache, our shoes are too tight, or the food being served in the cafeteria smells putrid, the way we detect, regulate and interpret those sensations helps us determine what actions we take. Overall, the results of these actions and associated feelings contribute to our sense of well-being, whether positive or negative.

Sensory processing is thought to have two main functions: protection and discrimination. Let's take a brief look at what these terms mean.

The Protective Function of Sensory Processing

Sensory processing is thought to help protect us from harm or danger. It has been linked to our fight, flight or freeze reactions and to the sympathetic and parasympathetic nervous systems (Ayres, 1972). The *sympathetic* system typically functions in actions requiring quick responses whereas the *parasympathetic* system functions with actions that do not require immediate reaction.

The complex functioning of the central nervous system seems quite abstract. Yet, neuroscientists and researchers can show evidence that sensory input causes physiological changes in the body. Both animals and humans use mostly touch, smell, and sound to detect danger. If a stimulus is processed as danger, our sympathetic system is activated and we prepare for "fight or flight." For example, if you smell something burning in your kitchen, your body immediately goes into protective mode. Your heart rate might increase, your breathing grows shallow, and you start to sweat. You start running around the kitchen searching for the source of the burning smell.

Conversely, sensory stimuli can have a calming effect, activating our parasympathetic nervous system, which, in simple terms, is responsible for regulating our body and maintaining homeostasis or a "feeling OK" state. Typically at a health spa, many forms of sensory stimuli are used to create a calm environment and provoke relaxation. For example, they play quiet, slow music and the staff talks in hushed tones. They might infuse calming aromas such as jasmine and lavender. And typically they provide warm towels, which are calming to the skin. All of these sensory experiences are designed to trigger the parasympathetic nervous system, thus having a calming effect.

The Discriminative Function of Sensory Processing

Each of the sensory systems includes a mapping component that supplies details for the central nervous system to consider. This is also known as discrimination. For example, when we touch (tactile) an object, the mapping function of the tactile system provides information about where the touch is occurring (the hand, not the back of the thigh) as well as whether the object is hard, soft, fuzzy, smooth, round, angular, and so on. Accurate information about these details helps us interpret the object in an effective and useful manner, whether it means to hold it without squishing it (if it is a ripe peach) or to grasp it firmly (as in preparing to serve a tennis ball).

Effective Sensory Processing

For many of us, sensory processing is effective and automatic. The typically developing nervous system involves ongoing, dynamic interplay between and comparison of information from all sensory systems. The outcomes of this process are seen in the responses we make to a given situation and reflect multiple contributing factors, including our individual sensory preferences as well as past experiences with certain sensations.

Even if we are able to process sensory information effectively, our interpretation of sensation is highly individualized. In other words, we all have unique sensory preferences. As a result, reactions to a given sensation (behavior) can be very different across people even when they experience the same sensory information. For example, you may love Mexican food, but your spouse finds it too spicy and upsetting to his stomach. Your brother likes loud rock-and-roll tunes, and you prefer soft classical music. Although each person's brain directs and is in charge of this interpretation, much of the process occurs at an automatic level without cognitive awareness of what is taking place.

It is beyond the scope of this book to give a comprehensive presentation of sensory processing. However, we will examine some of the components of the process in a simplified manner to provide understanding and insight into the behaviors you observe and thereby enable you to support individuals around you who have sensory challenges. The information that follows is an attempt to explain some of the components of sensory processing and how we can use that understanding to make "sense" of our own behaviors and those of others, including learners with HF-ASD.

As mentioned, sensory processing terms may vary from professional to professional, but most agree that effective sensory processing involves the ability to detect, modulate, interpret, and respond to incoming sensory input. So what does all of that mean? Good question! It can be very confusing at first. Let's take a simpler look at a few important aspects of sensory processing:

Technical Terms: *Detection, Registration, Neurological Thresholds*

Simplified Description: Sometimes we feel when a fly lands on our arm; at other times we don't. Sometimes background music is distracting and drives us crazy, and at other times we don't even notice it. Some of us love the smell of perfume and others are so bothered by the smell that they want to gag or run from the room.

The way we notice or tolerate different sensory experiences varies from person to person. For example, Joey loves to ride roller coasters – the more twists and turns the better! On the other hand, his brother Xavier grows queasy at just the thought of roller coasters. He prefers to keep his feet on the ground and play the carnival games. These two brothers have vastly different preferences for vestibular (movement) opportunities: One brother loves to move, and the other prefers sedentary activities.

To make matters a little trickier, our preferences don't always stay the same. What we like or what we can tolerate can change minute-by-minute depending on factors such as time of day, degree of stress, physical health, and level of hunger. For example, Barb almost always loves to listen to music really loud when she is driving in her car. However, on snowy days when driving causes her a lot of stress, it's a different story. At such times, her tolerance for auditory input is so low that she cannot tolerate any sounds in the car, let alone loud music. That is, her ability to tolerate auditory input is drastically changed due to the high degree of stress.

Each person has his or her unique sensory footprint, and each person becomes aware of sensory input at different speeds or levels. Some of us need more input to detect or notice a stimulus, and others are so sensitive that we require very little intensity to notice the same stimulus.

A ***neurological threshold*** is a term that refers to the point that has to be reached before our brain becomes aware of a sensation. It is the brain's "aha moment" – the instant that it notices the sensation. Some individuals have a very high threshold – they need lots of intense input to reach their threshold and thus notice the stimulus. Others have very low thresholds and require very little input to reach their threshold and notice the stimulus.

To illustrate, let's compare the "threshold" to a bucket. Imagine that everyone has a unique sensory bucket. At the top of your sensory bucket is an imaginary line. This is the "aha line" – the line that needs to be reached for the brain to notice a sensation.

Sensory buckets come in a wide variety of sizes. Some people have very large sensory buckets and need lots of sensory input to fill their bucket and reach the "aha

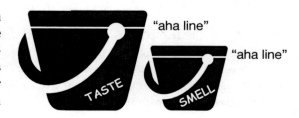

line." Others have very small sensory buckets and require very little sensory input to reach their "aha line," while yet others have sensory buckets that fall in between the very large and the very small.

In addition, it is possible for one person to have a small sensory bucket for one sense and a large bucket for another sense. For instance, Ali has a small sensory bucket for smell; he notices immediately when his teacher wears White Gardenia cologne. The scent causes his small bucket to quickly fill, and his aha line is reached easily. Thus, Ali notices the smell rapidly. At the same time, he has a large sensory bucket for taste; he can eat habañera peppers without reacting a bit. Even though habañera peppers have a really strong taste, he can easily tolerate the spiciness because his large sensory bucket can hold a lot more input.

Dunn's Model of Sensory Processing (1997) describes these neurological thresholds along a continuum. At one end of the continuum, we can be hyposensitive, or underresponsive, to sensory stimuli. This makes us less likely to detect the stimuli, or another way of looking at it, it means we need a greater intensity of input to reach our threshold and notice the stimuli. We have large sensory buckets. At the other end of the continuum, we can be hypersensitive, or overresponsive, to sensory input. This makes us more likely to detect the stimuli – we need much less intensity to detect the sensation. We have small sensory buckets. Figure 1.2 shows a threshold continuum.

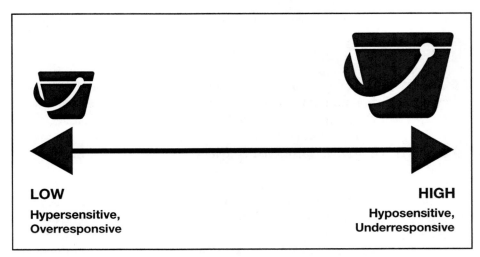

LOW   **HIGH**

Hypersensitive,   **Hyposensitive,**
Overresponsive   **Underresponsive**

Figure 1.2. Neurological threshold continuum.

Adapted from Dunn (1997).

Technical Terms: *Interpretation, Modulation, Arousal Levels, Self-Regulation*

Simplified Description: At any given point, an endless amount of sensory information is bombarding our brain, which then has to sort through the sensory chaos, pick out the important information, and ignore the rest. When sensory input enters our brain, the brain immediately interprets the sensation and sends us a message to either respond or not respond. The brain relates the incoming sensations to any similar past experiences we may have had. If we have previous experience with the particular sensation, it may evoke certain memories, emotions and/or reactions. For example, when Paul smells apple pie, it immediately evokes memories of his mother baking apple pie each year on his birthday when he was a young boy. Similarly, when Angelique hears the sound of her baby crying in the middle of the night, she immediately gets out of bed and goes to his room to check on him, as it usually means he needs her.

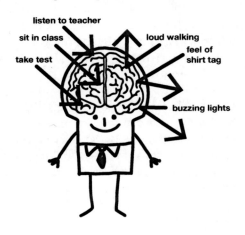

When the brain determines the need to respond to relevant sensory information, it helps match our reaction to the sensory event or situation at hand.

> Lizzie is crossing the street with her mother. All of a sudden she sees a speeding car and hears it beeping loudly. She screams and runs for cover with her mom. This is an appropriate response to the sensory input Lizzie received; it is a match. However, during free play in her preschool classroom, a student "zoomed" his car towards Lizzie, making a beeping noise with his mouth. Lizzie screams and runs for cover. This might be considered an over response to the sensory input Lizzie received: It was not a match.

> When Mattea hears a sound in the middle of the night, his "fight-or-flight" reaction is triggered, and his heart races, his breathing grows shallow, and his muscles tense. He yells for his mom to come to his rescue. Mattea's reaction to the sound that woke him in the middle of the night would be considered a match. When Mattea's mother starts to blow dry her hair several rooms away from where Mattea is playing, he

has a similar fight-or-flight reaction. His heart races, his breathing grows shallow, and his muscles tense. He yells for his mom to come to the rescue again. His response to the sound of the hairdryer might not be considered a match. His mother is puzzled by his extreme reaction to such an everyday sound.

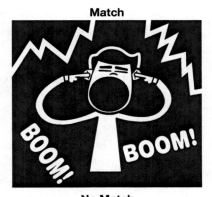

Match

The brain's ability to sort and respond to sensory input has a large impact on our ability to learn, move, and behave in a manner that is considered "socially typical" and, therefore, acceptable and effective. It also has a significant impact on our **arousal level** – a technical term used to describe how alert, energetic, and attentive we are at a given point.

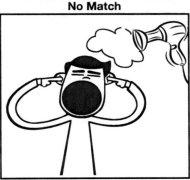

No Match

Our arousal levels fluctuate throughout the day. Sometimes our arousal level is elevated. We might feel energetic, bouncy, and active. At other times, our arousal level takes a dive.

We might feel sluggish, tired, and heavy. And sometimes, our arousal level falls in the middle. We might feel quiet, still, and focused. No matter what the situation, most of us strive for an "optimum level of arousal" (Mayes, 2000) – or homeostasis. That is, we aim to have an arousal level that is a match to the activity at hand, and we perform best when we are at this optimum state of arousal. If it is a match, our arousal level allows us to participate comfortably and successfully.

Most of us use a variety of sensory tools, or sensory input, both consciously and subconsciously, to adjust our arousal levels on a daily basis. For example, when you are sitting in a meeting and feel your arousal level dip, you might notice changes in your body (i.e., your eyes are droopy, your brain is fuzzy/sleepy, your body is heavy). This is an important meeting, and you know your boss, who is sitting across the table, is watching you. You realize that you need to "wake up" immediately, so you start fidgeting with your pen, sipping cold water, chewing on a mint, and shaking your leg up and down under the table. All of these sensory stimuli begin to increase your level of arousal. You start to feel more alert and focused. You enter into that optimum level of arousal again (and your job is saved!).

A technical term for this process is **self-regulation.** Your ability to use sensory input to adjust how you feel is a very important aspect of self-regulation.

If you can consistently match your arousal level to the activity at hand, you would be considered to have good self-regulation skills. For example, when sitting in a meeting, you can sit still in your chair and keep your brain focused on the person talking. Or when you are at a rock concert, you can dance and cheer loudly when the band plays your favorite song. Or when it is time to go to bed, you can easily unwind and fall asleep. These are all examples of adjusting your arousal level to match the activity – or in technical terms – they are examples of self-regulation.

Individuals who have all of the above sensory processing aspects intact are likely able to use sensory information effectively and may experience success in many areas of daily functioning. These individuals are often responsive to home routines, manage successfully in community settings, and are frequently viewed favorably by teachers at school and bosses at work. Typically, such individuals can:

- Continue their play or work in the yard without being bothered by the noise of the lawn mower, weed eater, or edge trimmer.

- Eat a variety of foods, although some preferences may be evident.

- Make their way through the crowd to find a place at the curb to wait for the parade to begin, without reacting to the close proximity of other people.

- Tolerate the singing and dancing of the staff at a restaurant.

- Finish their seatwork or deskwork despite the noises coming from outside the window.

- Sit still in a movie theater for the duration of a two-hour movie.

Difficulty With Sensory Processing

Sensory processing is invisible and develops automatically. It happens on a subconscious level – we don't need to think about it. For these reasons, sensory processing difficulties are easily overlooked or misunderstood. Until recently, we only had accounts, however powerful, from individuals living with these difficulties. Now we also have research that is starting to "prove" these difficulties exist (cf. Lane, Young, Baker, & Angley, 2010; Marco, Hinkley, Hill, & Nagarajan, 2011; Myles et al., 2007), which makes it all the more imperative to have a good understanding of sensory processing.

Pioneer and occupational therapist Dr. A. Jean Ayres began exploring the link between sensory processing and behavior in the 1950s. In her revolutionary book *Sensory Integration and the Child* (Ayres, 1979), she theorized that difficulty with sensory processing might result in a variety of social, emotional, motor, and/or functional problems. Ayres referred to these difficulties as sensory integration dysfunction.

Inspired by the work of Ayres, and using the tenets from her sensory integration theory, many professionals have since explored the impact that sensory processing, or more specifically *difficulty* with sensory processing, can have on behavior and function.

For example, what was previously referred to by Ayers (1979) as sensory integration dysfunction is now referred to as *sensory processing disorder* (SPD) (Miller, Anzalone, Lane, Cermak, & Osten, 2007). Simply speaking, SPD occurs when a person's daily life is hindered by difficulty taking in sensory information and making sense of it in order to respond as expected.

Given that there is a wide range of sensory processing preferences and abilities, it is not considered to be a problem until responses to sensory input significantly interfere with daily functioning.

> Madeline might find the sensation of having her fingernails cut to be irritating and uncomfortable. However, she has discovered that if she cuts her nails after a bath when they are softer, she can tolerate cutting her nails once a week. She still dislikes it, but she can get through the task. Although Madeline demonstrates difficulty with this particular sensation, she has adapted to it and is an otherwise happy and functioning child. She is not considered to have SPD.

> Chantal, a 5-year-old with HF-ASD, also strongly dislikes having her fingernails cut, along with having her hair washed and combed, and teeth brushed. Every night this routine becomes a battle between Chantal and her parents. Chantal becomes agitated and screams and cries throughout the self-care routine. Chantal's parents are frustrated and come to dread this time of day. By the time the routine is complete, all three of them are physically and emotionally exhausted. They try not to think about needing to do it all over again the next day, but it is inevitable.

> Unlike Madeline, Chantal is experiencing sensory processing difficulties that are greatly impacting her daily functioning. Not only is she

struggling to participate or complete self-care tasks, but her emotional well-being and social relationship with her family are also impacted. This may be an example of SPD.

Sensory processing issues are complex and intertwined. They do not conveniently fit into one category or another. Recognizing this challenge, Miller et al. (2007) proposed that there are three main categories or patterns of SPD:

- Sensory Modulation Disorder
- Sensory-Based Motor Disorder
- Sensory Discrimination Disorder

Miller and colleagues (2007) further separated each category into subtypes. This updated view of SPD does not suggest any changes in the assessment and treatment of sensory issues, as discussed in Chapters 3 and 4. Rather, these new diagnostic categories, described below, are offered in an effort to provide consistent terminology helpful for future understanding, research, and education of individuals with SPD.

Pattern 1: Sensory Modulation Disorder (SMD)

SMD occurs when somebody has difficulty adjusting her responses to sensory input. Often it is challenging for this person to maintain an emotional and attentional state that is considered socially typical.

SMD Subtype 1: Sensory Overresponsivity (SOR). Individuals with SOR respond rapidly to sensory input. They find sensory input to be intense, uncomfortable, and even painful. These individuals have small sensory buckets (see pages 14-15), so it does not take much input to fill their bucket and cause it to overflow or burst. It is thought that individuals with SOR have a low sensory threshold that is easily met and quickly exceeded by sensory input (Dunn, 1999).

The overresponsivity or, as it is sometimes referred to, sensory defensiveness, can occur in one sense (e.g., just auditory overresponsivity) or in multiple senses (e.g., overresponsivity to visual, auditory, and touch). To make matters trickier, overresponsivity can fluctuate depending on factors such as time of day, environment, and emotional state. That is, what seems to bother a person with SOR one minute may seem not to bother him the next. Individuals with SOR may be emotionally reactive. Sometimes they may seem rigidly in control – desperate to limit exposure to noxious input. Additionally, they may withdraw or go to great lengths to avoid certain sensory situations.

Research has shown that individuals with SOR have an exaggerated physiological reaction to sensory input (Schaaf, Benevides, Leiby, & Sendecki, 2013). In other words, their fight-or-flight response is intensely activated when they are faced with certain sensations, often resulting in extreme emotional reactions to seemingly minor input. It is important to remember that these atypical responses are not deliberate but are physiologically automatic.

> Jupiter, a 9-year-old boy with HF-ASD, has been sent to the principal's office 10 times, and school has only been in session for 1 week! During class, the teacher has been using team-building exercises to encourage the students to learn more about each other. A lot of these games are active and hands-on, requiring the students to move about the classroom and work in close proximity to each other.

> The students were having a great time – well, everyone but Jupiter. Seemingly out of nowhere, Jupiter would lash out at one of the other students, screaming, hitting, and/or kicking them. The teacher was alarmed and frustrated. The principal was furious, especially after multiple offenses. Jupiter was heart-broken and miserable. It wasn't until Jupiter's parents met with the school staff, including the occupational therapist, that they realized that Jupiter often had the same kind of reactions in similar settings.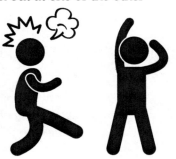

> The team began the process of a functional behavior assessment, interviewed Jupiter to gain his perspective, and conducted a sensory assessment to see if they could better understand his "behavior issues" and design interventions and support that could be helpful. Through this process, the team found that Jupiter was overresponsive to many sensations, including touch. The unexpected touch of another student brushing by him or grazing his arm when reaching for a nearby object sent him to full panic mode. All of the active and hands-on activities sent his system into a tailspin. He was in a constant state of fight-or-flight, ready to protect his sensitive body at any cost – even if it meant getting sent to the principal's office.

SMD Subtype 2: Sensory Underresponsivity (SUR). Individuals with SUR are slow to respond, or simply do not respond, to sensory information from the world around them. They seem oblivious, sluggish, or uninterested and, as a result, are frequently mislabeled as lazy. It is thought that individuals with SUR have a very high neurologic threshold for sensory input (Dunn, 1999). This means that they require a large dose of input to notice a sensation. Therefore, if a typical stimulus is presented, they may not detect it at all, thus appearing aloof, distant, etc.

> Taylor is now 15 years old. When he was in kindergarten, he was diagnosed with HF-ASD. While his cognitive abilities were always very strong, his social skills were often lacking. As a boy, he preferred to watch television or play a video game rather than playing outside with the other kids in the neighborhood. At school he had a hard time keeping up with his schoolwork, and mostly just sat on the bench reading a book at recess. When asked, PE was the class he hated the most. He did not like to do the exercises and had a hard time keeping up with the other kids when playing most of the games or activities during class time. As a result of his lack of activity, he was always a bit overweight, and he did his best to avoid most physical activities.
>
> Over the last couple of years, Taylor has become more active, has slimmed down, and made some new friends … thanks to Wii! His mother and his teachers have worked together to incorporate the Wii into his day both at home and at school. Taylor is motivated to do it, and it has helped to get his work completed. His social skills and interactions have improved as well, and now many of the other kids in his class and the neighborhood want to play the Wii games, too.

SMD Subtype 3: Sensory Seeking/Craving (SS). "Always on the go," that is the best way to describe individuals with SS for they are constantly striving to fulfill their seemingly limitless sensory needs. At times, they are reckless and invasive in their quest for sensory input. Not surprisingly, these sensory-seeking behaviors significantly impact their ability to function and participate successfully in daily activities.

It is easy to see why things may go awry. For example, the excessive and energetic attempts to gain sensory input may be highly distracting in a quiet classroom setting. These kids are labeled the "troublemakers" and spend lots of time "in trouble" for their behaviors. On the other hand, when forced to sit still and be quiet, they are not getting the input they need to regulate their arousal levels and may try hard to "hold it together," only to end up suddenly falling apart from the effort.

Some research suggests that people with SS have a high neurologic threshold and are actively attempting to provide input to reach this threshold and achieve regulation of arousal (Dunn, 1997). On the contrary, other research suggests that SS might not be solely a "meet my threshold" phenomenon, finding that not just any type of input is helpful in regulating these individuals. Rather systematic structured forms of certain input can be highly beneficial (Miller et al., 2007).

For whatever reason, people with SS seek immense amounts of sensory input.

Jacob is a 12-year-old boy with HF-ASD. For years, he's been getting in trouble for constantly being in motion. He can't sit still long enough to complete seatwork. He is always touching other people and objects. He bumps into other kids in the hallway. When playing at home with kids in the neighborhood, he's the kid who never wants to give up the swing to someone else because he can swing for hours. He rides his bike fast, up and down the street. Some say he's just a typical boy. His parents and teachers have called him "hyperactive." Jacob does not know how to explain his constant need for "more." He just knows he needs "more" …

more movement, more touching, more bumping, more crashing. At 12 years old, he tries to control his body, but it only results in a great deal of frustration. Jacob is a sensory seeker, and without proper support he may continue down this extremely frustrating path.

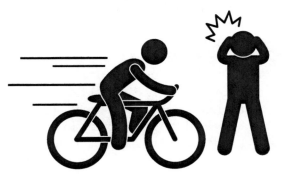

Pattern 2: Sensory-Based Motor Disorder (SBMD)

Due to poor sensory processing, individuals with SBMD may have poor ability to stabilize their bodies and/or move in a coordinated fashion. Their struggle with a variety of motor demands may impact their ability to complete even the most common daily tasks.

SBMD Subtype 1: Dyspraxia. Ayers (1972) defined dyspraxia as poor coordination of movement as a result of sensory processing difficulties. Individuals with dyspraxia often struggle with planning and carrying out an unfamiliar motor action. They appear clumsy and uncoordinated. Many have average intelligence and adequate muscle strength, but the problem lies in the "bridge" between their intellect and their muscles (Ayers, 1972).

Individuals with dyspraxia may be uncoordinated in terms of fine-motor skills and struggle with tasks such as writing, buttoning, and shoe tying. They may also find gross-motor tasks challenging, such as riding a bike and catching a ball. In addition, dyspraxia may affect their oral motor skills, making it difficult to speak clearly, blow bubbles, or drink from a straw.

Further, individuals with dyspraxia seem unsure of where their body is in space – almost as if they have a body full of Novocain – and are accident-prone. They tend to learn motor skills at a much slower rate than others. In fact, when attempting a new task, they often require a great deal of practice and repetition to achieve mastery.

> Richard, an 8-year-old with HF-ASD, struggled to keep up with his three brothers when playing active games. Although he could beat them at any quiet activity that required strategy and/or memory, activities involving any sort of movement brought on feelings of frustration and failure. No matter how many times he watched his brothers, Richard found it impossible to climb the rock wall on their playset, jump on their pogo sticks, and hit a baseball without using a tee. And he had completely given up on riding a bike. He could not figure out how to push the pedals, steer the handles, and use the brakes all the while trying to balance and not crash to the ground (which he did many, many times).

Richard has dyspraxia, which makes learning motor tasks very difficult. Eventually, without intervention, Richard might give up on these common childhood activities and stay on the sidelines watching his brothers have all of the fun.

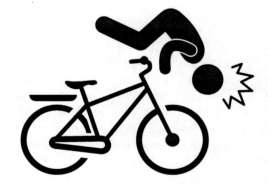

SBMD Subtype 2: Postural Disorders (PD). People with PD have difficulty maintaining a stable base of control and often appear droopy or weak. Postural control is important to help the body move against gravity. With good postural control comes support for the head, eyes and limbs during functional tasks. For example, when a person is standing on a stepstool reaching for a glass on the highest shelf, the postural muscles are actively working to provide support and balance so that the head and eyes can look up and the arm and hand can reach out and grab the glass.

> "Sit up, Dillen!" "Pay attention, Dillen!" "Are you listening, Dillen?" This is what Dillen, a 16-year-old with HF-ASD, heard on a daily basis at school. No matter how hard he tried, he could not stay seated upright during class for an entire day. His body felt so heavy and tired. Strangely enough, when he leaned on his arms or put his head down on his desk, he was able to pay attention so much better. It took all of his concentration to "sit up straight."

> Dillen knew that he was not making a great impression on his teachers when he slumped over, which made him anxious. No amount of social skills training, including discussion the importance of listening with his whole body, could change the fact that Dillen had very poor postural control. Only when the underlying sensory cause of his "slumping" is addressed will he experience greater success in this area.

Pattern 3: Sensory Discrimination Disorder (SDD). Individuals with SDD perceive that there is stimuli present and can regulate their response to that input; however, they have a difficult time interpreting the distinct qualities of the input. Incoming sensory information can be disorganized, fuzzy, and confusing. This makes it very difficult to determine the exact qualities of the information – and can be very frustrating. SDD can occur on just one sense or can impact multiple senses.

> Every time the teacher asked her students to retrieve an item from their desks, Rachael would slide off her chair, kneel down, and start pulling all of the contents from her desk onto the floor. This was very puzzling to the teacher, especially after she had specifically asked Rachael to stay in her chair and only remove the item requested.

Rachael had poor tactile discrimination, which caused her difficulty using her sense of touch to determine the item she was feeling when reaching in her desk. When she reached in her desk, everything felt similar, so to compensate she would use her sense of vision to look into her desk to try to find the object.

Summary

Now that we have discussed the many aspects of sensory processing, let's take a detailed look at the specific sensory characteristics of individuals with HF-ASD.

CHAPTER 2

HIGH-FUNCTIONING AUTISM SPECTRUM DISORDERS AND ASSOCIATED SENSORY CHARACTERISTICS

Another intrusion comes from loud noises and moving objects, which are, therefore, reacted to with horror. Tricycles, swings, elevators, vacuum cleaners, running water, gas burners, mechanical toys, egg beaters, even the wind could on occasions bring about a major panic. One of the children was even afraid to go near the closet in which the vacuum cleaner was kept. Injections and examinations with stethoscope or otoscope created a grave emotional crisis. (Kanner, 1943, p. 245)

_____

In what follows, I will describe a particularly interesting and highly recognizable type of child. The children I will present all have in common a fundamental disturbance which manifests itself in their physical appearance, expressive functions and, indeed, their whole behavior. (Asperger, 1944, p. 37)

With these words Leo Kanner (1943) and Hans Asperger (1944), respectively, began to describe the characteristics of children who have an autism spectrum disorder (ASD). This book focuses on a segment of the population, those who are referred to as "high functioning," who typically demonstrate:

- average to above-average intelligence
- social and communication deficits

27

- obsessive and narrowly defined interests
- concrete and literal thinking
- inflexibility
- challenges in self-regulation
- difficulties in understanding unwritten or unspoken rules
- health-related challenges
- problem-solving and organizational problems
- difficulty in discerning relevant from irrelevant stimuli
- behavioral issues, including anxiety, that are often related to lack of understanding stress or a defensive panic reaction (Asperger, 1944; Ben-Sasson et al., 2009; Buie et al., 2010; Endow, 2009; Groen, Zwiers, van der Gaag, & Buitelaar, 2008; Pfeiffer, Koenig, Kinnealey, Sheppard, & Henderson, 2011; Van Steensel, Bögels, & Perrin, 2011; Wing, 1981).

While there are exceptions to these characteristics within individuals with HF-ASD, we accept these traits as common to the exceptionality. Besides, although research has helped us understand HF-ASD, there is still much to learn (Aspy & Grossman, 2011; Reichow, Doehring, Cicchetti, & Volkmar, 2011).

Role of Differences in the Sensory System

One area that has received special attention in interventions for individuals with ASD in recent years is the sensory system. In fact, in the recently released DSM-5 (APA, 2013), sensory issues were included as a diagnostic criteria for ASD for the first time . We have strong evidence about the sensory differences inherent in ASD – both from a behavioral (cf. Lane et al., 2010; Myles et al., 2007) and a neurobiological standpoint (cf. Marco, Hinkley, Hill, & Nagarajan, 2011). Furthermore, according to extensive parent reports (Adamson, O'Hare, & Graham, 2006; Kern et al., 2008; Leekam, Nieto, Libby, Wing, & Gould, 2007) and autobiographical accounts by individuals on the spectrum (cf. Endow, 2009; Grandin, 1996; Shore, 2003), sensory differences are among the most problematic in HF-ASD.

Therefore, when assessing the behaviors of individuals with HF-ASD, it is of utmost importance to look at the behavior through a sensory processing lens; that is, consider the possibility that an underlying sensory processing difficulty is attributing to an observed behavior.

What follows is a brief description of the sensory areas as they relate to individuals with HF-ASD. Specifically, the following areas will be discussed in detail: (a) tactile, (b) vestibular, (c) proprioception, (d) interoception, (e) visual, (f) auditory, (g) gustatory, and (h) olfactory.[1] Each of these sensory systems will be reviewed in terms of four types of common sensory issues experienced by individuals with HF-ASD: overresponsivity, underresponsivity, craving, and discrimination difficulty. Specific observable behaviors are listed followed by a possible explanation for the behavior using a sensory processing lens. Finally, the discussion of each sensory system is accompanied by a look at the far-reaching emotional and behavioral implications of these sensory issues.

Tactile

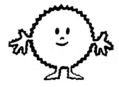

Of all of the senses, tactile differences, which are common in children with HF-ASD (Blakemore et al., 2006; Goldsmith, Van Hulle, Arneson, Schreiber, & Gernsbacher, 2006), present the biggest sensory challenges in daily living tasks such as dressing, tooth brushing, face washing, hair combing, and eating, according to parent reports (Reynolds & Lane, 2008). Tactile challenges also appear to be related to sleep disturbances (Shochat, Tzishinsky, & Engel-Yeger, 2009), and have been found to manifest themselves as behavior challenges, sometimes related to escape or avoidance (Güclü, Tanidir, Mukaddes, & Unal, 2007; Reynolds & Lane, 2008).

Hans Asperger (1944) also reported tactile problems in the children in his classic study. According to Asperger, "Many children have abnormally strong dislikes for particular tactile sensations, for example, velvet, silk, cotton, wool or chalk. They cannot tolerate the roughness of new shirts or of mended socks. Cutting fingernails is often the cause of tantrums" (p. 80). Around the same time, Kanner (1943) found eating problems in the 8 of the 11 children he reported on in his article "Autistic Disturbances of Affective Contact." He did not, however, specify etiology or correlation.

Individuals with HF-ASD may be overresponsive (overly sensitive) or underresponsive (not sensitive enough) to tactile stimuli. They may crave tactile input to such an extent that it impedes their ability to participate in meaningful activities. Or they may have difficulty differentiating different types

---

1 Often one behavior is caused by or related to more than one sensory processing area. For ease of understanding, each behavior here is attributed to the one sensory system that may often by the culprit.

or locations of touch. Each of these difficulties may bring with it a variety of problems that significantly impact daily functioning, general well-being, quality of life, and overall success.

Tactile Difficulties Seen in Individuals With HF-ASD

Tactile Modulation Difficulties

- Tactile Overresponsivity

- Tactile Underresponsivity

- Tactile Craving

Tactile Discrimination Difficulty

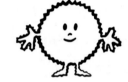

Tactile Modulation Difficulties

Tactile Overresponsivity
Individuals with HF-ASD who have tactile overresponsivity feel actual physical pain or discomfort when coming into contact with something seemingly minor. Therefore, when faced with a noxious tactile experience, they tend to react with strong emotions (fight) or escape at all costs (flight). This discomfort is often reported as heightened when the touch is unanticipated or sudden – like a person coming from behind and tapping your shoulder. Touching or being touched can be so distressing that a mere mention of or proximity to the noxious stimulus can cause a strong reaction.

Not surprisingly, therefore, individuals with tactile overresponsivity, also known as tactile defensiveness (Ayres, 1979), can appear anxious and hyper-vigilant, always on alert for the next tactile experience that may wreak havoc on their nervous system. In an effort to prevent or limit any uncomfortable tactile experience, they can be very controlling and rigid, often unwilling to accept change or try something new (Miller, 2006).

What You Might Observe	The Sensory Detective Says …
Child is hesitant to use glue, but the teacher convinces him to squeeze a drop or two on the art assignment. Suddenly, the child starts screaming and crying.	The child got glue on his hand, which was a painful sensation to him.
When the child enters the classroom and sees a bottle of glue on the art table, she starts crying and runs out of the classroom.	The child knows from past experience that touching glue is so bothersome that just the sight of the glue is enough to make her panic and run.
Child pushes or hits other students when standing in line.	The slightest light or unexpected touch from another student can set off a panic reaction. In order to protect his body, the child pushes or hits anyone who enters his "danger zone."
Child refuses to join games at recess and instead often just walks the perimeter of the playground by himself.	The child is so sensitive that the slightest touch from another person is an attack on his nervous system. He avoids any activity that involves close proximity to others such as football and tag.
Child grows aggressive at the end of each school day when it is time to walk to the buses.	The unpredictability of the bus is too much for the child to handle. There are far too many uncomfortable touch possibilities (e.g., someone brushes her arm when walking down the aisle of the bus), so just the thought of the bus pushes her over the edge. She will do anything to avoid the bus.
The child refuses to wear sneakers in gym class.	The child will only wear a certain brand of fur-lined moccasins. The annoying feel of any other type of shoe, including sneakers, sends her body into a tailspin.
Before wearing any shirt, the child insists on having not just the tag, but every piece of thread that attaches the tag, removed.	The feeling of the tag and threads on the back of his neck is so uncomfortable that he can't think of anything else until they are removed.
Despite being a high school junior, the child will only wear baggy sweatpants.	The feel of jeans on the child's skin is painful and sends his body into panic mode.
The child takes socks and shoes off constantly even when it is cold.	The child's feet are so sensitive that she cannot stand the feel of anything restrictive on her feet.
The child has a full-blown meltdown before bath or shower time.	The feel of the water splashing his skin is painful. Just the mere mention of the words "bath time" sends him into a full stress reaction.
The adolescent has severe underarm odor but refuses to wear deodorant.	The feel of deodorant on his underarm area is itchy and unbearable.
The teenager refuses to groom her bikini line hair before swim team practice.	The feel of a razor grazing her sensitive skin is agonizing, and she is so scared from past attempts that she even refuses to try any other option.

What You Might Observe	The Sensory Detective Says ...
The child gags when it is time to brush her teeth.	The sensation of the bristles brushing against her gums is nauseating. Just thinking about a toothbrush causes her to start gagging.
When his date suddenly reaches out to hold his hand, a young man blurts out, "Don't touch me!"	The unexpected touch was so uncomfortable that it set off his panic reaction. He automatically entered a "fight" mode, yelling at his date.

Tactile Underresponsivity

As opposed to overresponsivity, individuals with HF-ASD who have tactile underresponsivity may not feel or notice touch unless it is extremely intense. Consequently, they are often slow to respond to or notice certain forms of touch. These individuals may appear to be uninterested or to ignore others, but in reality they don't even notice the touch.

Tactile underresponsivity can cause safety concerns, when somebody commonly fails to even notice certain input that would register as painful to others. Often when individuals with tactile underresponsivity have scrapes and bruises, they have no idea when or how they occurred. Due to this low awareness of touch input, they may also have difficulties with regard to personal care and hygiene. For example, they might not notice food on their face or they might leave clothing twisted on their body. Many of us would 'feel' something is off and wipe the food or adjust the clothing. However, they do not realize the mistake, because they don't feel it.

What You Might Observe	The Sensory Detective Says ...
The child doesn't respond when teacher lightly taps him on the shoulder.	The child did not feel the light tap and, therefore, has no reason to respond. The teacher grows frustrated because it appears that the student ignored her.
Child has a huge scrape on his knee when returning from the playground, but he doesn't know how or when it happened.	The child took a nasty fall off of the slide but did not feel any pain. Therefore, he did not even check to see if there were any injuries. It was not a big deal to him, and he forgot it happened.
Child takes a bad spill during gym class but doesn't seem the least bit bothered.	The child failed to register a pain response even during a seemingly bad accident.
After lunch each day, the child has food on her face.	The child does not feel the food on her face and, therefore, has no reason to wipe it off.
Child frequently appears messy. At school, he typically has glue, marker and/or paint all over his arms and elbows.	The child does not feel the mess on his skin. Since he does not feel it, he does not realize that he looks messy.

What You Might Observe	The Sensory Detective Says ...
Child constantly wears her shoes on the wrong feet.	Although this might be uncomfortable to many, this child does not feel her shoes.
Child plays outside in the snow without shoes for 5 minutes before realizing he forgot to put shoes on.	Even with an intense sensation, like the coldness of snow, the child does not feel pain in a typical amount of time. It takes a longer duration of touch input for him to feel it.
Child is a constant safety concern because she does not respond to pain in a typical way (e.g., does not withdraw from scalding hot water).	The child does not immediately withdraw from a painful response such as hot water because it takes longer for her to feel the sensory input.

Tactile Craving

Individuals with HF-ASD with tactile craving can seem to be on a constant mission to touch everything and everyone in their environment. These children may especially love messy materials and may frequently be caught exploring items that are off-limits. In extreme cases, these individuals may seek tactile input that is harmful or dangerous. This can be scary and exhausting for caregivers, as they have to keep a vigilant watch over these children in order to maintain safety. With their need to touch others, tactile-craving individuals are often "space invaders," frequently intruding upon the personal space of others. This can be unsettling and can turn people off. This quest to fulfill a seemingly endless need for tactile input can significantly impact the ability to participate in meaningful activities and, therefore, has social, learning and safety implications.

What You Might Observe	The Sensory Detective Says ...
During seatwork, the child frequently bites areas of skin (e.g., fingers or arm), often so hard that it leaves teeth marks.	To try to maintain focus on the seatwork, the child seeks this very intense form of touch input.
When told, "don't touch that," the child manages to last about 3 seconds before reaching to touch it	Eager to please the teacher, the child tries hard not to touch the item but can't resist. His need to touch wins out.
The child refuses to leave the sensory bin area and has a meltdown when the teacher puts the lid on the bin.	The sensory bin provides a variety of touch opportunities, exactly what he is seeking. So when the teacher removes this highly desirable opportunity, it is distressing.
When completing art projects, the child is constantly playing with the glue, paint, etc. making a huge mess on himself and the surrounding furniture.	The feel of the messy materials is highly motivating to her, fulfilling her need for tactile input for the moment. The more time she has to play with the materials, the greater the mess, but the better the reward, so to speak.

What You Might Observe	The Sensory Detective Says ...
The child is constantly touching the students who sit next to him in class.	The child has a difficult time controlling his urge to touch everyone around him. Even though cognitively he realizes that it might be irritating, he just can't help touching those nearby.
The child repeatedly puts objects in the electrical outlets to feel the jolt.	The need for intense tactile input is so great, that the child takes excessive risks. Although extremely dangerous, the jolt from the outlet is the level of intensity he desires.
The child will touch or lean on everyone, even strangers in line at the grocery store.	The child cannot turn off his tactile-seeking behaviors, even in public. He gains the needed input by leaning on or touching anyone around.
The child takes a long time to complete any self-care activity such as bathing.	The need to touch is so great that she needs to stop and touch everything around her. This greatly interferes with her ability to stay focused on the task at hand, therefore, negatively impacting her efficiency and timeliness.

Tactile Discrimination Difficulty

Individuals with HF-ASD who have tactile discrimination difficulty cannot always determine the specific characteristics of touch input. For example, it may be difficult for them to know what they are touching without looking at the object. They might have difficulty distinguishing the texture or feel of what they are touching (e.g., sharp versus soft). They may have trouble identifying where they are touched without looking.

What You Might Observe	The Sensory Detective Says ...
When asked to find an item in his desk, the child frequently pulls all of the desk contents out and on the floor to search for the desired item.	When reaching inside the desk, the child cannot feel the difference between the materials (e.g., a pencil or a marker). Therefore, he needs to pull the items out so he can use his vision to find the object.
When searching for an item in her purse, the child needs to look in the purse to find it.	When she tries to search her purse with her hands alone, she frequently pulls out the wrong object. She needs to use her vision to find the desired object.
The child falls and scrapes his knee but insists on putting a bandage on his shin.	The child feels the pain but does not accurately feel the location of the pain.
When playing pin the tail on the donkey at a friend's birthday party, the child pins the tail on the wall a few feet down, despite being asked multiple times, "Are you sure your tail is on the poster?"	With his eyes covered, the child cannot determine the difference between the feel of the wall and the feel of the poster. Therefore, he cannot determine the surface area of the poster and is oblivious of placing the tail on the wrong surface.

Interoception

The little known but extremely important sensory system called interoception helps us to "feel" our internal state or conditions of our body. The interoceptive system brings in information such as pain, body temperature, itch, sexual arousal, hunger, and thirst. It also helps bring in information regarding heart and breathing rates and when we need to use the bathroom (Craig, 2003).

Numerous scientists believe that interoception is also a key component of our awareness of emotions. For many years, professionals have been debating the link between interoception and emotions. Research indicates that interoception, or our ability to interpret our internal body states, is the basis for how we view emotions (Craig, 2003). For example, say you are driving down the road and a car pulls out in front of you causing you to slam on your breaks and swerve to the side of the road, narrowly avoiding a collision. You might feel your heartbeat increase, your breathing get shallow, and your muscles tense. Based on how your body feels at that moment, you identify that you are scared. Given this link between processing interoceptive information and accurately sensing emotions, interoception becomes important in a variety of other related processes. For example, it has been found to be important to overall self-awareness, empathy, and other social cognition tasks (Craig, 2003).

Many individuals with HF-ASD have difficulties in the areas mentioned above, but only recently have researchers become interested in studying their interoceptive functions. Some preliminary brain imaging of individuals with HF-ASD has shown structural differences in the area of the brain responsible for processing interoceptive information (insula). Additionally, we have countless reports from both individuals with HF-ASD and their families of the differences they experience with interoceptive processing. These differences can cause a host of difficulties and struggles with even the most basic daily tasks. Furthermore, difficulties with interoception can cause significant problems with regulation. For example, if somebody does not effectively receive signals from their bladder, they may struggle in regulating their bladder functions. Or if somebody does not effectively receive signals regarding their heart rate, breathing rate, muscle tension, stomach status, and body temperature – all of which gives us clues about our current emotional state – they may struggle to regulate their emotions.

Interoception Difficulties Seen in Individuals With HF-ASD

Interoceptive Modulation Difficulties

- Interoceptive Overresponsivity

- Interoceptive Underresponsivity

- Interoceptive Craving

Interoception Discrimination Difficulty

Interoceptive Modulation Difficulties

Interoceptive Overresponsivity
Individuals with HF-ASD who have interoceptive overresponsivity may feel their internal states more readily. In fact, many times, they "over-feel" these internal states, causing them to be distracted by or highly anxious over certain sensations. For example, the sensitivity to interoceptive input may be so great that the seemingly minor stomach discomfort or a scratchy throat feels like a major health issue. At school, students may spend a lot of time visiting the nurse's office with a variety of discomforts and may miss a significant amount of school or work because they always feel sick.

Individuals who are overresponsive to interoceptive input may spend more time than typical in the bathroom, feeling extra sensitive to the urge to eliminate waste. This can be confusing to others. For example, when a student repeatedly asks to go to the bathroom during class, this can easily be misconstrued as avoidant behavior, when in actuality the smallest urge to urinate makes the student feel he needs to make a trip to the bathroom.

What You Might Observe	The Sensory Detective Says ...
Student requests bathroom breaks very frequently.	The child is extra sensitive to the urge to urinate or eliminate waste from his bowels. The slightest urge causes a feeling of discomfort or emergency.
Student visits the nurse's office several times a week complaining of aches, pains, and ailments.	The child overly feels internal states, and the slightest discomfort can feel like a major health issue.
Child limps on an injured ankle for weeks longer than expected.	The child continues to feel pain in the ankle even when it might seem almost healed to others.
During the winter, the student refuses to take jacket off when coming in from recess.	The child's awareness of body temperature is keen, and she feels cold much longer than the other students.
Child seems always to be hungry and/or thirsty.	The child might feel hunger or thirst much sooner than the other students. The smallest twinge of hunger or thirst may feel intense – like she hasn't had food or drink in days.
The child seems to panic after a short period of physical exertion.	The child may be very sensitive to the increase in heart rate and/or breathing. Such feelings can be uncomfortable and/or intense, causing the child to panic
The child is overly dramatic over a seemingly minor ailment (e.g., hangnail, runny nose, or stubbed toe).	To a child who is highly sensitive to his internal body states like pain, the feeling is amplified significantly.

Interoceptive Underresponsivity

As opposed to overresponsivity, individuals with HF-ASD who have interoceptive underresponsivity may not notice their internal body signals unless they are extremely intense. Consequently, they may not detect certain body states that may lead to significant difficulty with common, everyday tasks. For example, when individuals with HF-ASD are underresponsive to interoceptive input, they may not feel the urge to eliminate waste until the last minute when the feeling becomes very intense. This may cause frantic races to the nearest bathroom. In even more extreme situations, they may not recognize these sensations until it is too late, resulting in accidents. These difficulties cause very significant complications with toilet training.

This interoceptive underresponsivity can cause health-related concerns. For example, when individuals with HF-ASD are underresponsive to interoceptive input, they might not "feel" a sore throat or a urinary tract infection (UTI) and, therefore, not obtain or seek the medical care. Failure to treat certain illnesses can obviously be a serious matter.

Underresponsivity to interoceptive input can also make identifying stress and emotions difficult. Thus, many do not sense that they are experiencing a certain emotion until the body signals are very, very intense. This causes problems because, in order to have effective emotional regulation skills, it is important to recognize an emotion at a lower intensity level and start using a calming strategy before the emotion gets "out of control." Therefore, failure to sense an emotion until it is intense makes it difficult to use a calming strategy effectively. This is a common difficulty in individuals with HF-ASD – they struggle with identifying and acting on their emotions early, often resulting in explosions and/or meltdowns.

What You Might Observe	The Sensory Detective Says ...
When needing to eliminate waste, the child seems to wait until the last minute and then races to the bathroom.	The child does not effectively process signals from the bladder and/or intestinal tract and does not sense the need to use the bathroom until the feeling is very extreme.
The child is difficult to toilet train, having frequent accidents and never telling the adult that she needs to use the bathroom.	The child does not sense the urge to eliminate waste and, therefore, does not tell an adult that she needs to use the bathroom.
The child never seems to feel hungry and/or thirsty and almost has to be "forced" to eat or drink.	The child does not effectively process the signals regarding hunger and thirst and simply does not feel discomfort.
The child may have a fairly significant health issue but never complain of symptoms (e.g., strep throat, urinary tract infection, broken finger).	The child does not sense the discomfort in her throat, urinary tract, or finger and, therefore, does not report it.
The child has difficulty recognizing the early signs of an emotion and seems to have all-or-none emotions.	The child does not sense the subtle changes in his body, such as faster heart and breathing rate or tense muscles. He only senses these changes when they are at the extreme.
The child has difficulty using calming strategies effectively, so once he senses stress, it is often too late.	Once a child's stress/emotions are intense, it is often too late to use a calming strategy effectively. The key is to use the strategy at the start of the stress, when it is less intense.

Interoceptive Craving

Although the sense of interoception has been examined and discussed in other fields for years, only recently has interoception and the impact of corresponding sensory issues been considered in the field of autism. At this point, we do not know enough to comment on possible sensory craving behaviors in individuals with HF-ASD.

Interoceptive Discrimination Difficulty

Individuals with HF-ASD who have interoceptive discrimination difficulty cannot always pinpoint the exact feeling they sense from their internal systems. For example, they might have a general feeling of discomfort in the abdominal region but cannot distinguish if it is hunger or a need to use the bathroom. Or they might know that the cause of the abdominal discomfort is hunger but cannot determine the level of hunger (I can wait 30 minutes vs. I need to eat now!).

Because persons with interoceptive discrimination difficulty may have trouble detecting the differences in body states, it can make distinguishing between different emotions (mad vs. happy) or intensity of emotions (mildly angry vs. extremely angry) challenging. As a result, these individuals may report that their body feels similar whether they are really mad or really happy. Or they might be able to correlate certain body signals to feeling nervous but fail to notice the slight difference in body signals when feeling a little nervous vs. really, really nervous. An important part of emotional regulation is attending to and recognizing the subtle changes in one's body states and knowing what to do when experiencing those sensations. Not being able to identify these differences can make emotional regulation very difficult.

What You Might Observe	The Sensory Detective Says ...
When traveling, you ask the child if he has to stop to use the bathroom, and often the reply is, "I don't know" or "Maybe."	The child truly might not know if he needs to use the bathroom. He may have a general feeling of needing the bathroom but can't determine if he can wait or if it is an immediate need.
A child frequently complains of hunger, but when given food she only eats a bite.	The child may have mistaken the feeling of hunger for another body state, like needing to go to the toilet.
The child complains of feeling sick but can't express any specific symptoms.	The child may have a vague feeling of illness but can't pinpoint the feeling to specific areas or complaints.
The child insists that she is happy even though she clearly is angry.	The child might not be able to distinguish the subtle differences in internal body symptoms. For example, she realizes that her heart beats fast both when she is very happy and when she is very angry. However, the other body signals feel the same, making it difficult to distinguish between the two emotions.
The child can identify when he is angry but can't identify the degree or intensity of the anger.	The child has a general sense of the way his body feels when he is angry; however, he does not notice the slight difference in body signals when feeling a little angry vs. really, really angry.

Vestibular

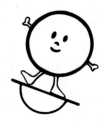

The vestibular system provides input to the brain about the body's movement through space and impacts movement, posture, balance, coordination of both sides of the body, eye movement, planning of motor movements and vision (cf. Devlin, Leader, & Healy, 2009). Research shows both vestibular overresponsivity and vestibular underresponsivity in learners with HF-ASD (cf. Kern et al., 2007; Vernazza-Martin et al., 2005). Indeed, individuals with HF-ASD can crave vestibular movement, so much so that it significantly impacts their daily lives. Problems related to the vestibular areas, such as posture (Molloy, Dietrich, & Bhattacharya, 2003) and orientation (Kern et al., 2007; Kern et al., 2010) also impact learning and functioning across home, school, and community.

Vestibular Difficulties Seen in Individuals With HF-ASD

Vestibular Modulation Difficulties

- Vestibular Overresponsivity

- Vestibular Underresponsivity

- Vestibular Craving

Vestibular Discrimination Difficulty

Vestbular Modulation Difficulties

Vestibular Overresponsivity
Individuals with vestibular overresponsivity tend to have a low tolerance for activities that involve movement. They may dislike movement and get very anxious and upset when asked to perform certain movement activities. Many times, individuals with HF-ASD who are sensitive to movement outright refuse to alter their body position or let their feet leave the ground. This is called "gravitational insecurity" (Ayres, 1979). Some children even lock their joints into a rigid position in order to stabilize their bodies and avoid sudden movement.

What You Might Observe	The Sensory Detective Says ...
The child cannot perform activities in gym class (i.e., doing a somersault).	The child may attempt this activity, but the fear of establishing a new position (particularly involving the head), the disorientation after moving into a crouching position, slowness in reorienting and pushing the body to do a somersault, would likely make this another uncomfortable experience.
The child does not complete work or work is sloppy.	The child may have difficulty copying from the board or may lose his place on the page.
The child has difficulty or does not attempt to put on socks and shoes and/or tie his shoes.	The feeling of bending down and moving the head into the position needed to reach shoelaces is so frightening that the child refuses to do any activity that requires bending over.
The child has a major meltdown every time a parent playfully spins or tips her upside down.	The child is so sensitive to movement that it triggers a panic response.
The child won't go on the equipment while playing in the park.	The child becomes anxious and/or nauseous when his feet leave the ground. He may be terrified by being tipped backward as he swings upward or forward as he swings back down. He may constantly feel that he is falling or being hurtled to the ground.
The child gets extremely upset when her hair is washed in the shower.	The child may panic at being bent backward when wetting or rinsing hair.
No matter how many times the child practices, he is very hesitant to use the escalator in the mall.	The movement of the escalator is unnerving to the child.

Vestibular Underresponsivity

Underresponsivity is observed in the child who swings or spins to such an extent that we, as sensory-typical individuals, fear that she will become dizzy or nauseated. However, many times these children can tolerate very intense movement without a single side-effect. Because they do not register typical levels of movement, individuals who are underresponsive to vestibular input do not get much pleasure from movement activities such as running, swinging, or climbing and, therefore, are drawn to more sedentary, quiet activities. Additionally, vestibular underresponsivity can lead to difficulties with balance, posture, and motor coordination, further leading these kids towards sedentary activities or activities that do not challenge their vestibular systems.

What You Might Observe	The Sensory Detective Says ...
The child does not use her hands to protect her body when falling.	The child may not feel the sensation of falling, thus not realizing the need for protection until well after the fall.
Even when all of his friends need a break, the child can spend all day riding the roller coaster without a break.	The child can tolerate very intense levels of movement activities.
During gymnastics class, the child has a very difficult time walking on the balance beam without stepping off the beam.	Because the child's vestibular system is not sensitive to small movements, the child does not notice the sensation of tipping quickly enough to adjust himself and stay balanced on the beam.

Vestibular Craving

Individuals with HF-ASD who crave vestibular input can appear to be in constant motion and are often usually described as "on the go." Some children crave so much movement that it seems almost impossible for them to "sit still." In extreme cases, they may seek extreme forms of vestibular input and take significant risks to gain the input they crave. This can include jumping from high places or dangling upside down from a piece of furniture. This can be scary and exhausting for caregivers, who have to keep a vigilant watch over these children to maintain safety. Further, this quest to fulfill a seemingly endless need for vestibular input can significantly impact the ability to participate in meaningful activities. That is, it has social, learning and safety implications.

What You Might Observe	The Sensory Detective Says ...
The child is in constant motion. Cannot seem to sit still during class time.	The child craves more and more movement because his brain is not interpreting the movement messages correctly.
The child is frequently getting in trouble at recess for doing dangerous tricks on the playground equipment.	The child takes extreme movement risks to meet his need for vestibular input.

Vestibular Discrimination Difficulty

Individuals with HF-ASD who have vestibular discrimination difficulty cannot always determine the specific characteristics of movement. For example, they may have difficulty knowing the direction in which they are moving or facing. It is especially challenging for them to know which direction they are moving when they close their eyes and cannot rely on vision to help guide their movements. In extreme cases, individuals with vestibular discrimination difficulty might not feel the difference between being upright vs. upside down or being tilted left vs. tilted right.

What You Might Observe	The Sensory Detective Says ...
During a game of pin the tail on the donkey, the child moves across the room in the opposite direction of the donkey poster.	The child knows he is moving across the room but does not realize that it is in the opposite direction from the poster.
When playing touch football with friends, it is challenging for the child to quickly switch directions to avoid getting tagged.	The child struggles to feel the difference between moving right and moving left, which makes changing directions quickly a huge challenge.

Proprioception

Little receptors in the muscles and joints send messages to the brain that help us move, sit, hold items, and balance. These receptors, or proprioceptors, allow us to move without having to think about what our body is doing. For example, our proprioceptive system allows us to sit down in a chair without looking and helps us to "know" that we are pulling our shirt on correctly with- 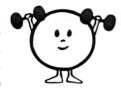 out looking in the mirror. This system also helps us keep our balance when walking; it helps us "right ourselves" when we are carrying heavy objects, and it helps us to automatically know how much force to use with our movements. "Motor planning" is a term that is often used in this context; it refers to the planning and execution of a series of movements, which most of us do routinely without thinking about it.

But for some children with HF-ASD, these movements are not automatic. Research on proprioception and autism is equivocal. Weimer, Schatz, Lincoln, Ballantyne, and Trauner (2001) found deficits in the proprioception system of learners on the spectrum. Conversely, Fuentes, Mostofsky, and Bastian (2011) reported of their study participants "... despite demonstrating motor and sensory impairments, the ASD group showed no impairments on all tested proprioceptive tasks." They further stated, "It is still possible, however, that there exist autism-associated differences in the ... integration of proprioceptive information" (p. 1359). Yet another study found an overly strong proprioception system in individuals with autism and suggested using this system to teach social and related skills (Mostofsky & Ewen, 2011).

In the absence of more conclusive research, we turn to countless personal reports of the movement and coordination difficulties experienced by individuals with HF-ASD. Such difficulties are partially due to a poorly functioning proprioceptive system and can include overresponsivity (overly sensitive), underresponsivity (not sensitive enough), craving, and discrimination difficulty.

Proprioceptive Difficulties Seen in Individuals With HF-ASD

Proprioceptive Modulation Difficulties

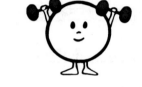

- Proprioceptive Overresponsitivity

- Proprioceptive Underresponsitivity

- Proprioceptive Craving

Proprioceptive Discrimination Difficulty

Proprioceptive Modulation Difficulties

Proprioceptive Overresponsitivity
Individuals with HF-ASD who are overresponsive to proprioception may find firm touch to be extremely uncomfortable and they might dislike activities that provide strong input into joints like running, jumping, hopping, skipping, or climbing. When required to endure an unpleasant activity, they react with strong emotions (fight) or try to escape at all costs (flight).

What You Might Observe	The Sensory Detective Says ...
When a parent attempts to take the child to a new gymnastics class, the child has a full-blown meltdown in the lobby of the gymnastics center.	The child is so adverse to even the potential of a movement activity that it triggers a panic response.
The child spends every outdoor recess sitting alone on a bench looking at Pokémon cards.	The child avoids any active games or activities at recess because they are very uncomfortable to him.
The child wants to sleep without blankets even on cold nights.	The pressure from the blankets is distressing to the child.

Proprioceptive Underresponsivity

As opposed to overresponsivity, underresponsivity to proprioceptive input may cause difficulty feeling or sensing one's muscles and joints. The sensation can be likened to having a full-body shot of Novocain. Imagine trying to move when your entire body is essentially numb.

Individuals who are underresponsive to proprioception are uncoordinated and have significant difficulty performing motor tasks in an automatic fashion. Typically, our proprioceptors send information to the brain about movements that we commonly perform, and the brain takes this information and forms memories of these common movements (e.g., signing your signature, bringing a spoon to your mouth, throwing a ball). Then, when we do engage in these common movement activities, we call on the memory of the task so that we don't have to really "think" about performing it, but can complete it automatically. However, individuals who are underresponsive do not always develop these movement memories, which wreaks havoc on their ability to perform everyday tasks in an efficient and easy manner. For example, climbing a set of stairs becomes a major chore because at each step they have to stop and "think" about each leg and foot movement as they progress up or down.

What You Might Observe	The Sensory Detective Says …
The child is very slow when going up and down stairs and needs to look at his foot placement on every single step.	The child does not "feel" his feet and legs and has to rely on vision to help him move up and down the stairs.
The child has difficulty copying from the board and is typically the last one finished in class.	The child does not have reliable motor memory for the formation of each letter and has to think about how to write each individual letter. Therefore, this task can take a long time.
The child frequently has bruises but doesn't know how she got them.	Lacking awareness of where her body is, the child is accident prone, frequently bumping into objects.
The child slumps over on desk during seated work.	Because movement and maintaining positions can be such a chore, the child grows tired and slumps over and/or leans on his arms and hands for support.
The child loves to sing in the church choir, but when dancing or gestures are involved, he is always a few beats off, and his movements do not quite match those of the other singers.	Difficulty sensing arms and legs makes it difficult for the child to move them in a rhythmic or timely fashion, especially when combined with another task such as singing.

What You Might Observe	The Sensory Detective Says ...
The child is extremely slow to get dressed in the morning, causing a great deal of family tension.	Performing even daily tasks is a major chore for the child who has difficulty feeling and coordinating her body. She is not motivated to complete these tasks when it causes such frustration, and when coupled with her parents urging her to hurry, the result is a high degree of tension every morning.
The child can only fall asleep when surrounded by huge body pillows and heavy blankets.	The inability to feel her body, coupled with the fear of falling out of bed (because that has happened way too many times), the child can only relax enough to fall asleep if she has the pillows and blankets grounding and securing her body.

Proprioceptive Craving

Individuals with HF-ASD who crave proprioception tend to be "bumpers and crashers." They seem to have an unlimited need for activities that provide a lot of pressure into the joints and muscles. These children can be rough and physically intense in their play, which may be a turnoff to other children. Furthermore, they may accidentally break toys and other materials due to the amount of force they crave. Indeed, the need for proprioceptive input can be so great that the child will "bump and crash" with little regard for safety. Not surprisingly, this quest to fulfill a seemingly endless need for proprioceptive input can significantly impact the ability to participate in meaningful activities.

What You Might Observe	The Sensory Detective Says ...
The parent frequently catches the child climbing tall pieces of furniture and jumping to the ground.	The child enjoys intense forms of proprioception and takes excessive risk to fulfill this need.
The child constantly breaks his pencil.	Because he craves intense proprioceptive input when writing, the child pushes the pencil into the paper so hard that the pencil tip breaks.
The child repeatedly puts objects in the electrical outlets to feel the jolt.	The need for intense proprioceptive input is so great that the child takes excessive risks. Although extremely dangerous, the jolt from the outlet is the level of intensity he desires.
The child touches or leans on everyone, even strangers in line at the grocery store.	The child cannot turn off his proprioceptive-seeking behaviors, even in public. He gains the needed input by leaning on or touching anyone around.
Every day after school, the child jumps back and forth between couches and chairs for 2+ hours.	Especially after trying to keep her body under control at school, the child craves even more intense proprioceptive input. It sometimes seems like her need cannot be satisfied by any amount of activity.

What You Might Observe	The Sensory Detective Says ...
The child is constantly kicking the back of the desk of the classmate in front of him.	The child has a difficult time controlling his need for proprioceptive input. Although the child knows that the kicking is bothersome, he just cannot turn it off.
The child sleeps with 10 blankets piled on top and pillows surrounding her body.	The child relies on the heavy proprioceptive input provided by the blanket and pillows and can only fall asleep with this extreme form of pressure.

Proprioceptive Discrimination Difficulty

Individuals with HF-ASD who have discrimination issues cannot always determine the position of their body or judge the amount of movement or force needed for a particular activity. For example, when playing catch, the child might not be able to judge how hard to throw the ball resulting in them over or under throwing the ball.

What You Might Observe	The Sensory Detective Says ...
The child constantly slams doors.	The child overshoots the energy needed to close the door, resulting in slamming.
The child frequently breaks glasses and dishes when unloading the dishwasher.	The child misjudges the force needed to carefully stack plates or set glasses in the cabinet.
The child adamantly avoids eyes-closed activities.	The child relies on his vision to compensate for the inability to judge exactly where his body is in space. Therefore, eyes-closed activities can be very disorienting and upsetting.
When playing "Simon Says," the child is typically a little off when imitating a body position.	The child is unable to determine if her body position is an exact match to that of the leader.
The child's handwriting is very light and difficult to read.	The child does not accurately judge the amount of pressure needed to write legibly.

Visual

Compared with other sensory areas, the visual system appears to be a relative strength for children and youth with HF-ASD. For example, Dunn, Myles, and Orr (2002) found that almost half of the 42 children they studied responded to visual input similarly to those who had no special needs. Fewer than 20% had definite visual-related problems, and an additional 19% were likely to experience difficulties in this sensory area. Because there is a need for more research in this area, controversy exists as to whether learners on the spectrum have increased acuity (Ashwin, Ashwin, Rhydderch, Howells, & Baron-Cohen, 2009; Tavassoli, Latham, Bach, Dakin, & Baron-Cohen, 2011).

Visual problems related to sensory processing can take many forms. Children and youth with HF-ASD may be underresponsive to visual input. Frequently they cannot find what they are looking for. They appear not to see the social studies book in their desk that is "right there on top of the science book." They cannot find the can of corn in the pantry that is "right before their eyes," or they don't see the green T-shirt they are supposed to wear even though it is folded neatly in the dresser drawer.

However, these same children may be overresponsive to visual input and be able find a needle in a haystack or Charizard in a mess of 150 Pokémon cards. Why the discrepancy? Ashwin and colleagues (2009) have issued a call for a search for possible mechanisms underlying enhanced perceptual functioning and attention to detail seen in individuals on the spectrum. Others (Takarae, Luna, Minshew, & Sweeneys, 2008) have suggested that challenges may be related to difficulties related to perceiving movement. Still others have discussed the "sensitivity to local features embedded in more complex patterns" (Falkmer et al., 2011, p. 816). Motivation and concentration may also be related to the seemingly contradictory performance. It may take the child with HF-ASD tremendous concentration to focus on finding what he needs. When motivation is high, that concentration can be applied for short periods of time, but such concentration may be very tiring and require so much effort that it cannot be sustained easily for long periods of time.

Visual Issues Seen in Individuals With HF-ASD

Visual Modulation Difficulties

- Visual Overresponsivity

- Visual Underresponsivity

- Visual Craving

Visual Discrimination Difficulty

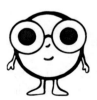

Visual Modulation Difficulties

Visual Overresponsivity

Individuals with HF-ASD who have visual overresponsivity may be able to see very fine details that others never notice. For example, they may immediately recognize a piece of furniture or a small picture frame that is moved out of place ever so slightly. Also, because they are so sensitive to visual input, they may experience discomfort and anxiety in the presence of certain irritants. For example, they might find bright sunlight to be painful or a classroom lit by fluorescent lighting to be distracting and bothersome.

What You Might Observe	The Sensory Detective Says ...
The child wants to wear sunglasses even when indoors.	The child is sensitive to all forms of light. The lighting, especially brighter lights (e.g., sun and fluorescents), can cause significant discomfort and anxiety.
The child grows irritable when playing outside on a sunny day.	While many children are in good spirits when playing outside on a sunny day, the child who is very sensitive grows irritable from having to endure the discomfort caused by the bright sunlight.
The child constantly puts his head down on his desk during class.	The fluorescent lights in the classroom are bothersome, and the child is seeking relief by shielding his eyes.
The child is distracted in classrooms with lots of pictures and posters on the walls.	The child is extra sensitive to visual clutter. The posters and pictures seem brighter and bigger to him and, therefore, more difficult to ignore.
The child refuses to open the blinds in their bedroom.	Sunlight is bothersome to the child, so she keeps the blinds closed to avoid the distress.
The child does not make eye contact.	Due to his sensitivity, looking at another person's eyes or face can be extremely uncomfortable and awkward.

Visual Underresponsivity

Contrary to those with overresponsivity, individuals with HF-ASD who are underresponsive to visual input may seem oblivious to visual items in the environment. For example, they may have difficulty "seeing" an item that they are looking for even if it is right in front of them. This is often baffling and frustrating to teachers and caregivers.

What You Might Observe	The Sensory Detective Says ...
The child's handwriting is sloppy and unorganized.	The child does not notice the lines of the paper and, therefore, does not use them as boundaries to help organize the appearance of his writing.
The child has difficulty dodging a ball during a game of dodge ball.	The child does not see the ball is coming toward him until it is too late.
The child does not recognize that another person is upset.	The child does not visually detect the facial expressions and body language of the person who is upset.
When the teacher uses a classroom hand signal to gain control of the students, the child with HF-ASD does not follow suit. The teacher always has to call the student's name and ask him to quiet down like the rest of his classmates.	It takes the child a long time to recognize the visual input, and by the time she does, it is too late. The teacher is already frustrated and is verbally requesting that he follow suit.
Despite looking in the mirror several times before leaving for school, the child typically has toothpaste on his face, a messy hairdo or a mismatched outfit.	When looking in the mirror, the child does not recognize all of the little details, such as a messy face, hair, or outfit.

Visual Craving

Individuals with HF-ASD who crave visual input seem to enjoy intense visual activities. They are frequently drawn to items that are bright, lighted, and/or fast moving and may watch these items for very long periods of time. They may also spend hours in front of a screen – be it a TV, computer, or video game.

What You Might Observe	The Sensory Detective Says ...
The child will only play with toys that have bright, blinking lights.	Because the child craves intense visual input, she only plays with toys that fulfill this need.
The child stays awake all night playing video or computer games.	The child craves the visual input provided by the screen of the TV or computer. The craving is to the point that it starts interfering with his daily activities.
The child constantly twirls a small string within his line of vision.	The child enjoys watching the movement of the string in all different directions and patterns.

Visual Discrimination Difficulty

Individuals with HF-ASD who have visual discrimination difficulty cannot always distinguish the differences when looking at different items. For example, they may find it hard to learn the letters of the alphabet and frequently reverse similar letters such as *d, p, b,* and *q.* They might also have difficulty determining subtle difference in facial expressions leading to poor recognition of others' emotions.

What You Might Observe	The Sensory Detective Says ...
When a parent asks the child to find a can of kidney beans in the pantry, he returns with a can of black beans.	The child was close but did not detect the subtle differences between the labels on the can.
Despite studying for hours, the child frequently fails her spelling tests.	The child does not naturally see the differences in the way words are spelled, causing great difficulty on spelling tests.
The child frequently asks others, "What is wrong?" or "Are you OK?" even if they do not show signs of being upset.	The child compensates for his difficulty reading the subtle differences in face and body language by continually asking others about their current state.
Even when prompted to check a certain word or sentence for errors, the child does not notice reversed letter(s).	The child does not automatically detect the differences between many letters, which causes her to reverse or write letters incorrectly.

Auditory

Research shows that individuals with HF-ASD do not process auditory information the same way as their nondisabled peers, showing both patterns of overresponsivity and underresponsivity (Källstrand, Olsson, Nehlstedt, Sköld, &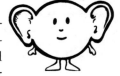
Nielzén, 2010; Kwon, Kim, Choe, Ko, & Park, 2007; Rosenhall, Nordin, Brantberg, & Gillberg, 2003). Problems are related to auditory processing rather than traditional hearing problems. That is, they typically have intact hearing abilities but may not efficiently or accurately interpret auditory information.

Summarizing his case studies of individuals with autistic psychopathy, Hans Asperger (1944) wrote, "There is hypersensitivity to noise. Yet the same children who are distinctly hypersensitive to noise in particular situations, in other situations may appear to be hyposensitive. They may appear to be switched off even to loud noises" (p. 80). The ramifications are profound. Those who experience sounds differently may avoid them or block them out, or they may seek out intense sounds that are not typical of most experiences. In either case, they may not be receptive to the type of auditory information that is necessary to learning social/relationship skills as well as the other building blocks necessary for a high quality of life. It is essential, therefore, to understand auditory issues in order to structure effective interventions (Marco, Hinkley, Hill, & Nagarajan, 2011).

Individuals with HF-ASD can have a number of auditory difficulties that compound their already chaotic world. They may be overresponsive (overly sensitive) or underresponsive (not sensitive enough) to sounds; they may crave auditory input so much that it impedes their ability to participate in meaningful activities; or they may have difficulty differentiating different types or location of sounds. Each of these difficulties can bring with it a variety of problems that significantly impact an individual with HF-ASD.

Auditory Difficulties Seen in Individuals With HF-ASD

Auditory Modulation Difficulties

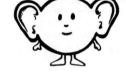

- Auditory Overresponsivity

- Auditory Underresponsivity

- Auditory Craving

Auditory Discrimination Difficulty

Auditory Modulation Difficulties

Auditory Overresponsivity

Some children with HF-ASD are so sensitive to certain sounds that they cover their ears, run away from a noise, or avoid loud environments at all costs. A seemingly typical noise, such as the school bell ringing, can be so intense for them that it causes pain. Such sensitivity to sound can cause a high level of stress and anxiety, and recent studies show that certain exposure to certain aversive sounds can activate the fight-or-flight response (Chang et al., 2012).

But it is not only loud noises that can be bothersome. Even gentle sounds can be highly irritating or distracting and prevent some children from being able to concentrate. They cannot listen to someone talk with the television on in the other room. In class, if other children are talking or even whispering, a child with HF-ASD may not be able to read or complete a worksheet.

What You Might Observe	The Sensory Detective Says ...
The child has a meltdown during every fire drill.	The sound of the fire alarm is so loud to the child that it causes physical pain and panic.
Throughout Fire Awareness Month, the child is constantly "obsessing" over the next fire drill. The child cries and screams every morning before school and frequently asks the teacher when the next fire drill will take place.	The sound of the fire alarm is so excruciating that just the mere thought of an impending fire drill keeps the child in a state of constant anxiety.
The child complains about the buzzing sound in the classroom, but the teacher is puzzled because she does not hear a "buzzing" sound.	The child is so sensitive that not only can he hear the buzzing noise of the fluorescent lights, he grows irritated and cannot concentrate because of it.
The child screams and holds his hands over his ears even before the fireworks start.	The loud booming of the fireworks are too much for the sensitive child to handle.
The child can hear the sound of an airplane way before the rest of the family notices the sound.	The child's hearing is so sensitive that he is able to notice sounds that others do not notice until they get closer or louder.
When driving in the car, the child screams, "Turn the music down!!! Too loud!!!" even though the music is fairly low.	Sounds are more intense to a child that is overresponsive. This heightened sensitivity can make even the slightest sounds too much to bear.

Auditory Underresponsivity

As opposed to those with overresponsivity, individuals with HF-ASD who are underresponsive to sounds may not notice sounds unless they are very intense, or they may notice the sound, but it takes them a lot longer than others to do so. These individuals may appear uninterested in or oblivious to things happening around them. They may appear to ignore others, but in reality they don't even notice the sound of someone calling their name or talking to them.

Parents and teachers often report that their children and students do not respond to them, even when there is no background noise. This failure to notice important sounds, such as a peer calling their name, a parent asking a question, or a teacher giving directions, can greatly impact an individual's success socially, both at home and at school.

What You Might Observe	The Sensory Detective Says ...
The child does not respond when the teacher calls his name.	The child is so undersensitive to sound that he does not detect the noise of the teacher's voice calling his name.
The child sleeps through the sound of the alarm clock even though it is right next to her head.	Even the loud noise of an alarm clock placed in close proximity to the child's head is not intense enough for the child to respond.
The child talks with a loud voice at all times.	Speaking in a loud voice sounds like a typical volume to the child who is underresponsive to sounds.
The parent has to give the same direction several times until the child is able to follow through with an otherwise easy task.	The child does not detect the parent's voice on the first few sets of directions. It is not until the parent gives the direction the fourth time that the child realizes that a direction was given.

Auditory Craving

Individuals with HF-ASD who crave auditory input may enjoy loud or constant sounds. Noises that seem to be irritating or distracting to many people are pleasant and helpful at meeting their need for intense noise. In an effort to meet their seemingly insatiable appetite for noise, individuals who crave auditory input may not only crave noises from other objects but may serve as the source of the sound themselves. That is, often these individuals are the loudest persons in a room, speaking constantly in a loud voice and/or constantly making noises (e.g., humming, singing, drumming their fingers).

What You Might Observe	The Sensory Detective Says ...
No matter how many times the teacher asks him to stop, the child constantly hums and drums his fingers on the desk during class.	The child seeks this form of auditory input to maintain focus in the classroom.
The child cannot complete her homework unless the TV or radio is on in the next room.	The child craves constant noise. In order to complete homework she needs the background noise of the TV or radio.
The child's parents are constantly asking her to turn down her music.	The child needs the music to be loud in order to gain the input she craves.

Auditory Discrimination Difficulty

Individuals with HF-ASD who have auditory discrimination difficulty cannot always distinguish subtle differences in sounds, which can greatly impede their ability to follow and understand spoken language. For example, they may find it challenging to detect the difference between similar-sounding words or have difficulty determining where a sound is coming from. These issues can present a constant struggle as the world around can sound like a confusing jumble of sounds and noises.

What You Might Observe	The Sensory Detective Says ...
When the teacher announces that indoor recess is over, the child is almost always the last student to clean up.	When multiple sounds are present in the classroom, like the teacher talking, a pencil sharpener buzzing and a nearby student laughing, the child cannot screen out and determine that the teacher's voice is the important sound on which to focus.
Although his mother is extremely patient, the child does not realize that she is upset until she is loudly yelling at him.	The child misses all of the subtle changes in his mother's voice when she is only a little upset. It is only when her voice changes significantly that he realizes that she is really angry.
The child cannot rhyme words.	The child has a difficult time hearing the subtle differences between words such as *cat, bat, rat*.
The child has difficulty attending to, understanding, or remembering what is said or read.	Because the child may be unable to attend she may need directions to be repeated and may only be able to understand and follow simple or two-step directions.
The child seems always to be confused about what to do next.	The child listens to the teacher's directions, but every other word sounds like a jumble. Therefore, it takes her a long time to figure out what the teacher asked and by then the class has moved on to the next direction.
The child does not understand sarcasm.	The child does not pick up on the subtle changes in a person's tone of voice when using sarcasm. Therefore, it is completely lost on him.
The child does not look in the correct direction of a person calling her name.	The child has a difficult time figuring out the location of sounds.

Gustatory

The gustatory or sense of taste is another area that can be difficult for children and youth with HFASD, leading many to (a) avoid certain tastes that are otherwise typical of children's diets, (b) eat only food with certain tastes, and/or (c) be picky eaters (cf. Bennetto, Kuschner, & Hyman, 2007; Blakemore et al., 2006; Reynolds & Lane, 2008). Asperger (1944) found similar characteristics, "There is often a preference for very sour or strongly spiced food, such as gherkins or roast meat. Often there is an insurmountable dislike of vegetables or dairy product" (p. 80).

Feeding difficulties are estimated to occur in as many as 70 to 90% of children with ASD (Cermak, Curtin, & Bandini, 2010). Using a sensory perspective, a child's reasons for choosing or avoiding certain foods often make perfect sense. For example, if the child is overresponsive to tastes, the food may be truly unpleasant, overpowering, or nauseating. On the other hand, if the child is underresponsive, the food may seem bland and unappetizing. Being unable to taste the food can be an unsettling prospect.

Feeding difficulties may also occur if a child seeks high amounts of gustatory input as he may crave strong tastes and even overeat due to a constant search for taste input.[1]

Gustatory Difficulties Seen in Individuals With HF-ASD

Gustatory Modulation Difficulties

- Gustatory Overresponsivity

- Gustatory Underresponsivity

- Gustatory Craving

Gustatory Discrimination Difficulty

Gustatory Modulation Difficulties

Gustatory Overresponsivity

Individuals who are overresponsive to tastes may find many foods to be highly unpleasant and offensive, which, in turn, can cause them to have very restrictive diets. Due to these limited diets of many children with HF-ASD, often consisting of only a few favorite foods, ensuring proper nutrition can be a concern. For example, a diet of chicken fingers, macaroni and cheese, and potato chips clearly does not provide the nutrition that a growing child needs. Therefore, in many cases, it is helpful to enlist the support of a nutritionist and an occupational therapist to systematically introduce foods that are tolerable and provide the nutrients that a child needs.

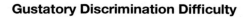

1 For the purpose of simplicity, feeding difficulties are only discussed under the gustatory sensory system. However, feeding difficulties may also be caused by other sensory issues. For example, tactile issues (i.e., the feel or texture of food), olfactory issues (i.e., the smell of the food), or interoceptive issues (i.e., not feeling hungry or full) may all contribute to feeding problems.

What You Might Observe	The Sensory Detective Says ...
The child only eats five foods, and eats the same five foods every day.	The child chooses a limited number of very specific foods that do not upset his sensitive sensory system. The longer he continues to have only a small repertoire of foods to choose from, the more rigid his food choices become.
The child who loves macaroni and cheese has a full-blown meltdown when his mom buys a different brand of macaroni and cheese.	Even though there is very little difference in brands, because his sense of taste is so sensitive, the child finds the new brand of macaroni and cheese repulsive. Just the thought of eating the new brand sends the child into full-blown panic mode.
The child cannot successfully eat at restaurants with her family.	The child is so highly sensitive and picky that she cannot deviate from her standard diet and try to find something similar to her standards on the menu. The family has firmly encouraged her in three restaurants, all resulting in a meltdown.

Gustatory Underresponsivity

Contrary to those who are overresponsive and find many tastes to be over-powering and strong, individuals who are underresponsive find many foods tasteless or bland. As a result, they might not taste and enjoy the flavors of food in the same way that others do or they may be drawn to foods with strong, robust flavors. The underresponsitivity to taste can also cause diffi-culty in sensing if a food is spoiled or just does not taste typical.

What You Might Observe	The Sensory Detective Says ...
The child accidentally eats spoiled food, not realizing that it tastes bad.	We know that milk is bad because it tastes sour, so we stop drinking it. The bitter taste of medication tells us that it's not candy. If a child doesn't receive those signals at all, or at a high enough level to sound an alarm, he's in danger of eating or drinking things that can make him sick.
The child can eat an entire jalapeño or other spicy food without a flinch.	Being undersensitive to tastes, the child can easily eat strong foods that typically taste very spicy or bold to others. The child might report not even tasting the strong food.

Gustatory Craving

When persons with HF-ASD crave gustatory input, they tend to be in con-stant search of items to put in their mouth. For example, they will seek out bold flavors, whether sweet, salty, spicy, minty, or sour. They may also have a tendency to eat frequently and/or overeat. Some even use non-food items to gain the gustatory input that they crave.

What You Might Observe	The Sensory Detective Says ...
The child constantly licks and mouths food and non-food objects.	The child is on a constant mission to gain the tastes he is craving. He has little concern for safety or hygiene when "tasting" non-food objects.
The child is always chewing strong-tasting mints or gum.	The child is seeking high levels of taste input, and the strong mints and gum fulfill this need.
The child frequently overeats.	The act of tasting and eating is so fulfilling to the child that it becomes difficult to stop at a healthy point.

Gustatory Discrimination

When a person has difficulty with gustatory discrimination, determining the exact qualities of food from a taste perspective can be difficult. Therefore, these individuals may be unable to determine the difference between tastes, especially if they are flavors that are relatively similar (e.g., a cherry vs. strawberry lollipop).

What You Might Observe	The Sensory Detective Says ...
The child has difficulty determining if a food is a little spicy or really, really spicy.	To this child most spicy foods taste the same, and he cannot taste the difference in the levels of hotness or spice.
When provided with two similar food items (e.g., an orange and a grapefruit), the child can not rely on taste alone to accurately identify them (he needs to look at the items to correctly identify).	The child has poor discrimination and cannot taste the different qualities in these two fruits.

Olfactory

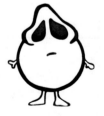

Our olfactory system is constantly bombarded with smells. In fact, most of us are unaware of the extent to which smells exist in the environment and how important our ability to process this input can be to our well-being. The olfactory or sense of smell also presents challenges to many individuals on the autism spectrum. Thus, studies have reported both odor identification deficits (discrimination) as well as a heightened sense of unpleasantness of odors (Bennetto et al., 2007; Hilton et al., 2010; Hrdlicka, 2011).

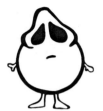

Olfactory Difficulties Seen in Individuals With HF-ASD

Olfactory Modulation Difficulties

- Olfactory Overresponsivity

- Olfactory Underresponsivity

- Olfactory Craving

Olfactory Discrimination Disorder

Olfactory Modulation Difficulties

Olfactory Overresponsivity

Not being able to block out the countless smells in the environment can be overwhelming and distracting. For example, some people experience physical distress when faced with insulting smells – often smells that others around them hardly notice at all. People with HF-ASD may experience one or all of these difficulties when they are overresponsive to olfactory information.

What You Might Observe	The Sensory Detective Says ... 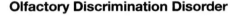
Every time the teacher tries to sit next to the child in order to give her 1:1 support, the child grows angry and screams, "Get away from me!"	The teacher's aftershave is so overwhelming to the child that it causes her panic. The child does not intend to hurt the teacher's feelings. She is just protecting her sensitive sensory system.
The child becomes very upset and sometimes even gags when visiting his aunt's home.	Although seemingly subtle and pleasant, the child does not like the smell of the air freshener used by his aunt. The smell is so offensive to him that it causes him to gag.
The child adamantly refuses to eat in the school cafeteria.	The smell of the cafeteria is so unpleasant to the child that even the thought of eating there causes a strong emotional response.

Olfactory Underresponsivity

If an individual with HF-ASD is underresponsive to olfactory information and perhaps does not notice smells, it can have significant impact on safety, health, and hygiene. Smells can serve as an important sign of danger. For example, smelling smoke can serve as a signal to search for fire. Or smelling a pungent scent coming from food can serve as a signal that the food is rancid.

Smells can also serve as hygiene clues. Generally speaking, if a person senses that she is giving off an odor, such as foul-smelling armpits or bad breath, it serves as a clue to shower or brush teeth. However, when somebody is underresponsive and does not notice these smells, they miss the signals and clues and, therefore, might not take desirable action.

What You Might Observe	The Sensory Detective Says ...
When his mother accidentally burns a bagel in the toaster, the child reports that he does not smell the strong odor.	The child does not detect the smell of burning or smoke. This can be dangerous as the smell of smoke can be a first alert to a fire.
The child does not shower every day even after exercise.	The child is undersensitive to the smell of her body odor and does not realize that she smells offensively.

Olfactory Craving

Some individuals with HF-ASD seek olfactory input to the point that it interferes with their ability to successfully participate in activities within the home, school, and community. It may seem strange to others if somebody is constantly holding items to their nose, or if they surround themselves with scents, like air fresheners and perfumes, it can be overwhelming or even off-putting to others.

What You Might Observe	The Sensory Detective Says ...
When sitting in class, the child frequently leans close to girl in front of him and sniffs her hair.	The child craves the smell of the shampoo used by the girl.
The child uses way too much perfume.	The child loves strong smells so she puts on a lot of perfume in order to gain the strong smell she craves.
During art class, the child smells everything he can get his hands on and is so distracted by smelling objects that he misses the information presented by the teacher.	The child cannot turn off his need for olfactory input, and the art classroom is full of unique items to smell.

Olfactory Discrimination Disorder

When a person has difficulty with olfactory discrimination, he may struggle to accurately identify a particular scent or even determine the source of a smell.

What You Might Observe	The Sensory Detective Says ...
The child is unable to correctly identify an object based on smell (e.g., lemon vs. lime) alone.	The objects may smell so similar that the child has a tough time determining which object is which.
The child accidentally sprays mint mouth spray on as cologne and does not realize the mistake.	The child does not recognize the difference between a minty scent and a cologne scent.
The person notices a putrid smell coming from the refrigerator but struggles to determine the source of it.	Although the person can smell the spoiled food item, determining the exact smell is tricky (e.g., is it spoiled milk vs. a rotten lemon?).

Hopefully, the preceding sections helped to clarify how an observable behavior may be due to one or multiple sensory issues. Many times, sensory issues have far-reaching implications and may attribute to extreme responses and very difficult moments not only for the individual with HF-ASD but also for those who love, support, or teach them. The following section highlights these behavioral and emotional responses to sensory stimuli.

Behavioral and Emotional Responses to Sensory Stimuli

A well-regulated sensory system helps us to know what information to attend to and what information to filter out to maintain a state of homeostasis (cf. Hilton et al., 2010; Myles et al., 2004). Challenges related to the sensory system have a tremendous and often negative impact on the behavior, social functioning, and daily living experiences of children and youth with HF-ASD. For example, Blanche and Schaaf (2001) used the term "proprioceptive seeking" to define a behavioral pattern consisting of hyperactive and "aggressive" or unsafe and impulsive behaviors that may stem from children's search for increased sensory input.

A relationship also exists between social challenges and sensory impairment, particularly in the areas of tactile and olfactory. For example, a common aspect of an intimate relationship is close proximity and touching (kissing, hugging, etc.). If a person is overresponsive to touch and smells, this can cause extreme discomfort when involved in the "typical" activities of an intimate relationship.

The same is true for how a learner on the spectrum reacts to multisensory stimuli – the input of multiple incoming sensations. Tasks invoking multi-sensory responsiveness include difficulty paying attention, problems concentrating, getting lost easily, seeming oblivious in an active environment, making needs known in sensory-unfriendly environments, and recognizing and responding to the needs of others (Dunn, 1999). Similarly, Baker, Lane, Angley, and Young (2008) found a relationship between behavior and emotional problems and multiple sensory areas, including being underresponsive to sensory input and seeking/craving sensory input.

Sensory challenges impact functioning in all environments, including family life. In fact, parents' responses to items under this category on the *Sensory Profile* (Dunn, 1999) indicated that this is the greatest area of concern for children and youth with HF-ASD (Dunn, Myles, & Orr, 2002; Schaaf, Benevides, Leiby, & Sendecki, 2013). For example, a substantial number of children and youth with HF-ASD frequently or always:

- seem anxious
- display emotional outbursts when unsuccessful
- demonstrate poor frustration tolerance
- are sensitive to criticism
- cry easily

In addition, they:

- don't tolerate change in plans, expectations, and routines
- are inefficient at accomplishing tasks
- don't perceive body language and expressions correctly

Parents and teachers also report that these children:

- have difficulty making friends
- need more protection from life's events than others (Dunn et al., 2002).

Schaaf et al. (2013) examined the effects of sensory differences on family daily routines, reporting six major areas in which sensory issues in autism impacted daily life:

1. **Flexibility.** Family members reported needing a high degree of flexibility to accommodate the needs of their children with ASD. Their children's difficulty to regulate their behavior in the face of sensory insults causes caregivers to be extremely adaptable. For example, they cancel plans, delay plans, take multiple vehicles to an event, vacuum when the child is not home, cook only meals that do not smell unpleasant to the child, attempt to ensure that siblings interact in a way that does not negatively impact the child, and so forth.

2. **Familiar vs. unfamiliar.** Families spend a considerable amount of time creating routines that provide structure to minimize the assault on the sensory system of their children with autism. Routines at home are relatively easy to structure; experiences in the community can be more difficult. For example, department stores, grocery stores, the home of others, all present challenges and families often limit these activities.

3. **Difficulty completing family activities.** In general, parents perceive that families who have a member on the spectrum have greater difficult engaging in family activities than those who do not have a child with autism. Meltdowns related to the sensory impact of "getting ready" activities, such as getting ready for school or getting ready for bed, are frequent occurrences. Sensory issues and need for movement also create problems at mealtimes, especially dinner. Air travel, sightseeing, long car rides, going out to dinner, and attending sporting events all present sensory challenges to the learner on the spectrum. As a result, planning often includes extensive modifications to limit sensory influence and potential meltdowns related to sensory issues.

4. **Impact on siblings.** Sensory challenges also impact siblings. Because caregivers spend extensive amounts of time attempting to meet the sensory needs of their children with autism, they report not having enough time with their other children. Two-parent families try to divide their time among their children, but families acknowledge that their child with autism was the first priority.

5. **Need for constant monitoring.** Caregivers are vigilant – always on alert for sensory violations. "All of the caregivers in this study expressed the feeling that they could rarely divert their attention from the child, because of the child's intense needs for sensory stimuli, as well as adverse reactions to other sensory stimuli" (Schaaf et al., 2013, p. 383). Monitoring occurs on two levels: the environment and the child. Caregivers are constantly searching the environment to ensure it is sensory-friendly. They also are continually watching the child carefully, looking for signs of sensory distress in order to prevent tantrums, rage, and meltdowns related to sensory elements in the environment.

6. **Strategies to improve family participation.** Parents/caregivers report having a high level of awareness of sensory demands in all environments and adjusting demands whenever necessary to ensure that their children can participate in a variety of activities. Strategies include developing routines, having a variety of sensory supports on hand, and flexibility on the part of caregivers.

A picture of the child with HF-ASD is emerging. This is a child who, although working hard, may not complete his work. He cannot tell whether his teachers or parents are pleased or upset with him. When changes occur in his environment, his already anxious state intensifies, leading him to cry, scream, tantrum to express his frustration, or "withdraw." He wants to have friends, but he doesn't understand their social language. In this intense emotional state, he may demonstrate behaviors or coping strategies that are more typical of younger children since they are most familiar and may have been successful in the past. He is extremely gullible with peers, particularly those who have recognized a potential vulnerability. This may lead others to engage in bullying, teasing, or practical jokes to elicit what is perceived as a humorous or entertaining reaction. Such peers can also lead the child to break rules as he does not understand the social ramifications.

This child has tactile issues. He doesn't understand the concept of space and feels uncomfortable standing in line or being too close to others – at school, at the bank, in the grocery store. This creates more anxiety. He has problems writ-

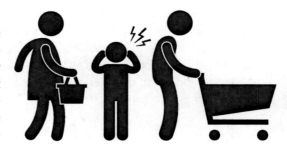

ing. In addition to fine-motor problems, the sound of the pencil writing on paper is grating to him. Visual and vestibular problems are also evident. He has difficulty copying from the chalkboard, and he is fatigued because in order to face someone, he needs to move his entire body toward them and concentrate – hard. In addition, the proprioceptive system causes difficulties. He wants to do his work in the beanbag chair at the back of the room, but since there is only one, it is not always available. He can't seem to concentrate unless he is in the beanbag chair or lying on the floor. He has auditory problems and doesn't process what the teachers or parents say, or does so very slowly. He may not respond right on time or do what he is supposed to do. Yet, when asked to repeat back what was said, he is able to do it verbatim. When his teacher makes a comment about his attention, he is not sure what she meant. Was she upset? Was she teasing? He is constantly on the alert for a noise that is painful for him – he fears the fire alarm and the static noise made by the intercom system before an announcement in the grocery store. To cope, he sometimes tunes it out. He seems oblivious to everything going on around him. When his teacher gets his attention, he doesn't know how long he was "gone" or what he missed. He also doesn't know how to get the information he missed in the meantime. His visual sense may be the strongest, but he may still have trouble finding the social studies book in his desk and he may have difficulty concentrating if the lights are too bright or too dim.

Finally, add in gustatory and olfactory problems. He is particularly stressed by gym and lunch, which occur right after each another. Gym is a problem because of all the smells. Just thinking about them upsets him. Lunch is another challenge. He forgot his sack lunch, and the food in the lunchroom tastes like sandpaper; the smell of the lunchroom is even worse. He is hungry but knows that the food will likely make him gag. What can he do to get food that he likes?

If you were the child with HF-ASD and had some or all of these challenges, how would you act or react? How long would it take before you exploded? Or withdrew?

Considering how much children and youth with HF-ASD have to tolerate on a daily basis, it is no wonder they sometimes resort to tantrums, rage, or meltdowns, but as we will see in Chapter 4, we can help restructure their environment to reduce or eliminate sensory issues. But first we will discuss how to assess sensory issues in Chapter 3.

ASSESSING SENSORY PROCESSING ISSUES

Children and youth with high-functioning autism spectrum disorders (HF-ASD) display a variety of complex behaviors across academic, behavioral, social/emotional, leisure/recreational, and vocational areas. Each of these areas may be impacted by sensory processing issues. As we have seen in the previous chapters, sensory problems are variable and can occur inconsistently, interfering with performance at home, school, and community. In addition, these behaviors can be sporadic, occurring on one occasion and not on another, even when the circumstances appear to be identical.

Sensory difficulties can be impacted by a variety of variables that may include:

- amount of structure present
- task requirements
- personality of adult involved
- level of stress
- changes in routine
- method of instructional delivery
- amount of rest
- level of abstraction

Additional variables may be specific to individuals or the situations in which they are involved. To determine possible causes and solutions to these otherwise puzzling behaviors and reactions, teachers and parents must become "sensory detectives."

All of these variables make the assessment of sensory issues challenging. Simply using one checklist for one observation in one environment will likely not yield accurate information. In order to develop intervention strategies that will support the child across various settings and situations at home and at school, we must try to understand the behaviors we observe. Accurate and effective assessment of an individual's sensory needs requires thorough examination of the child and her environments.

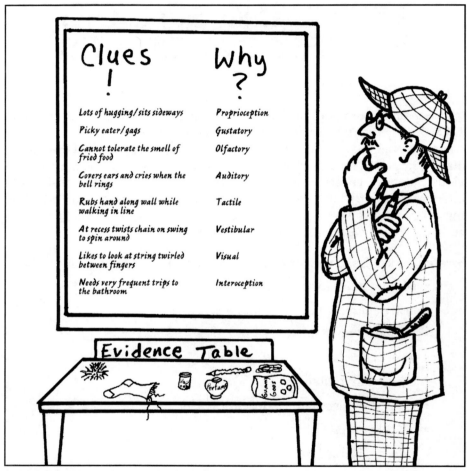

Figure 3.1. Sensory detective at work.

Table 3.1 lists the classic considerations that can support effective assessment. We realize that time constraints and staff availability may preclude you from addressing each of these considerations. Collaboration among various adults in the child's many environments is one way to address assessment in a more timely fashion.

Table 3.1
Techniques and Suggestions for Evaluating Individuals With ASD

1. Assess individuals across a variety of settings (e.g., recess, music, social studies, lunchroom). A series of brief assessments that represent students' environments is preferred to one lengthy observation in one environment.

2. Observe students in the presence of different individuals (e.g., teachers, peers, parent).

3. Examine student behavior under varied task demands (i.e., independent activities, written work, group work, unstructured activities).

4. Observe students at different times of the day (i.e., morning, afternoon, before or after lunch).

5. Seek information from multiple respondents (i.e., teachers, parents, paraprofessionals, ancillary staff, peers).

6. If possible, assess students in a variety of potentially stress-invoking scenarios (i.e., an unexpected change in routine, instruction with a high level of verbal content, academic demands above instructional level, presence of a substitute teacher).

7. Consider the environmental or assessment setting as a critical component for understanding the student's behavior (i.e., proximity of student to teacher, desk arrangement, lighting, noise levels).

8. Talk to the student. Some insights may be gleaned by just asking the right questions.

9. Consider the value of observation during other assessments. Observing the student during intelligence or achievement testing can provide valuable insights and assist in selecting the appropriate sensory assessment.

10. Look for patterns as well as differences of performance across multiple variables. These can provide valuable insights for developing interventions.

Adapted from Lowrence, L. (1994). *Techniques and suggestions for evaluating persons with autism.* Paper presented at the meeting of the Autism Society of America Convention Kansas City, MO.

Assessment Tools

Although neuroscientists are learning more and more about sensory issues and behavior, we are not yet able to determine definitive cause-effect relationships. Current "best practice" in assessment techniques reflects this growing knowledge in the neurosciences and its application to sensory processing in everyday life.

A variety of instruments provide valuable information about sensory processing, which are summarized in Table 3.2. These measures may be categorized as formal and informal. Formal assessments include norm-referenced and standardized instruments that compare an individual's profile to those of typically developing peers. Informal assessments, on the other hand, consist of reviews of records, inventories/checklists, interviews, and observations. Informal assessments often provide descriptive information about behaviors and can be useful in developing strategies that address those behaviors. However, they do not yield developmental scores for comparison with a normative population. Unlike most formal assessments, informal tools are usually easy to administer, are inexpensive, and do not require specific training to be conducted. Occupational therapists (OTs) typically have a foundation of understanding about sensory processing and can administer and interpret sensory processing assessments.

Guide to Instruments to Assess the Sensory Areas

The Texas Autism Resource Guide for Effective Teaching or TARGET (http://www.txautism.net/target-texas-autism-resource-guide-for-effective-teaching) provides information on sensory assessments. TARGET provides a brief narrative on each measure along with tables that indicate (a) the age range for which the measure is appropriate, (b) method of administration/format, (c) approximate time to administer, (d) subscales and types of scores yielded, and (e) a description of the research conducted on each tool.

Table 3.2
Formal and Informal Assessment Measures

Title	Author	Year	Administration Time	Age Range	Who Can Complete the Tool	Who Can Score/Interpret the Tool
Sensory Profile	Dunn	1999	30 minutes	3-10	Parent or familiar caregiver	OTs, professionals with a strong foundation in sensory integration and sensory processing theory
The Short Sensory Profile	McIntosh, Miller, Shyu, & Dunn	1999	10 minutes	3-17	Parent or familiar caregiver	OTs, professionals with a strong foundation in sensory integration and sensory processing theory
Adolescent/Adult Sensory Profile	Brown & Dunn	2002	15-30 minutes	11+	Self-report or report of familiar caregiver if individual unable to complete independently	OTs, professionals with a strong foundation in sensory integration and sensory processing theory
Infant/Toddler Sensory Profile	Dunn	2002	15-20 minutes	7 months-36 months	Parent of familiar caregiver	OTs, professionals with a strong foundation in sensory integration and sensory processing theory
Sensory Profile: School Companion	Dunn	2006	15-20 minutes	3 to 11 years 11 months	Child's teacher	OTs, professionals with a strong foundation in sensory integration and sensory processing theory
Sensory Integration and Praxis Test (SIPT)	Ayers	1989	2-3 hours for all 17 subtests: (10 minutes per subtest)	4 through 8 years 11 months	Professionals trained and certified in sanctioned SIPT administration and interpretation courses	Test must be submitted to publisher for scoring or be scored on pre-sold computer disks. Interpretation is included with scores
Sensory Processing Measure (SPM)	(Home Form) Parham & Ecker (School Forms) Miller-Kuhaneck, Henry, & Glennon	2007	15-20 minutes	5 to 12 years	Parent and/or teacher rating scale	OTs, professionals with a strong foundation in sensory integration and sensory processing theory
Sensory Processing Measure– Preschool	(Home Form) Miller-Kuhaneck, Henry, & Glennon	2010	15-20 minutes	2 to 5 years	Parent and preschool teacher/daycare provider	OTs, professionals with a strong foundation in sensory integration and sensory processing theory

Informal Assessment Measures

Title	Author	Year	Administration Time	Age Range	Who Can Complete the Tool	Who Can Score/Interpret the Tool
Sensory Integration Inventory-Revised	Reisman & Hanschu	1992	30 minutes	Children and adults	Parent, teachers, others familiar with the child	OTs, professionals with a strong foundation in sensory integration and sensory processing theory
Sensory Screening in Building Bridges Through Sensory Integration	Yack, Sutton, & Aquilla	2003	20-45 minutes	Not specified	Parent, teachers, others familiar with the child	OTs, professionals with a strong foundation in sensory integration and sensory processing theory

Guidelines for Observation

In addition to administering formal and informal measures, direct observation of the learner with HF-ASD in her many environments can provide insight into the learner's sensory challenges. Specifically, direct observation analyzes the child's behavior, the tasks in which she participates, and the environment in which she is asked to perform. Kienz and Miller (1999) developed the Questions to Guide Classroom Observations to guide teachers, therapists, or others familiar with sensory systems in observing a child in the classroom setting (see Table 3.3.). A series of 38 questions address the following areas: (a) child, (b) task, (c) physical environment, (d) social context, and (e) cultural context. Results of this observational assessment can yield information about sensory processing and its impact on a child's ability to perform expected activities in the classroom. It is most often used in conjunction with other formal or informal measures.

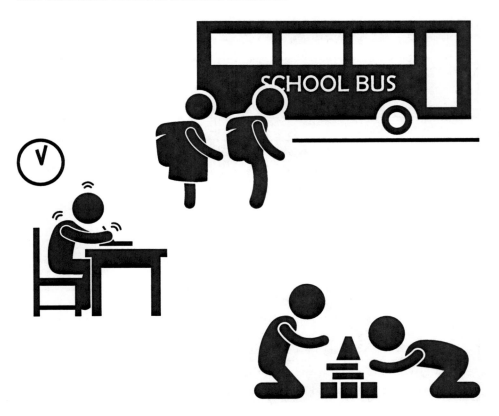

Table 3.3
Questions to Guide Classroom Observations

Variable	Questions
Child	What are the child's strengths and difficulties in terms of motor skills, cognitive skills, communication, play and praxis?
	What methods does the child use to communicate? What are the child's preferred modes of interaction?
	Does the child imitate others? Does the child make eye contact? Does this fluctuate? In what way?
	What does the child enjoy or seek out?
	What are the child's specific behavioral concerns? When do they occur?
	What calms or arouses the child?
Task	What is required? Expected?
	How do others complete the task?
	Is the task clear and understandable? Is the task predictable?
	Does the task have a clear end? How does the child know when it is completed?
	Does the task have a clear sequence? How many steps are there? How are instructions provided?
	Is assistance available? What type? What materials are used?
	What are the sensory properties of the task and materials? How long is the task?
Environment and Context	
Physical	What is the spatial arrangement of the area?
	What is the size of the area?
	Which objects and people are present? How is the area organized?
	How easily can the child move within the area? What is the temperature?
	What is the noise level?
	How densely packed are people and objects? What time of day is it?
	What odors are present? What is the lighting source?
	How visually stimulating is the area?
Social	Who is with the child?
	With whom does the child choose to interact? Who encourages the child's best performance?
	What form of interaction occurs with peers? Teachers? Other adults?
Cultural	What is expected within this environment?
	Are the expectations or rules of the environment clear? How are rules communicated?

From Kienz, K., & Miller, H. (1999, March). Classroom evaluation of the child with autism. School system. *Special Interest Section Quarterly*, 6(1), p 4. Used with permission by Therapy Association, Inc., PO Box 31220, Bethesda, MD 20824-1220.

Interpretation

Interpretations of assessment measures are largely instrument dependent and are most often made by occupational therapists or other professionals trained in understanding the sensory systems who are skilled in administering, scoring, and interpreting this type of information. Skilled interpretations provide a comprehensive look at the child across environments, under various settings, with different adults and peers, and so on. In all cases, these individuals must be careful not to go beyond the intention of the instruments.

To be useful, recommendations that stem from an assessment must be detailed enough to be implemented by the many staff members and parents who have contact with the child. The information will help teachers and parents develop programming strategies that support the child's success in various environments.

> Assessment revealed that Jon has vestibular issues that appear to impact his ability to sit still and attend. As a result, at his IEP meeting, his teachers and parents discussed strategies that would address these needs. They thought that a Disc 'O' Sit™, an inflatable disc, or camping pillow would provide Jon with the needed vestibular input and help him sit in his chair and pay attention.

Close collaboration among the occupational therapist and other team members in implementing the recommendations is essential to ensure that (a) recommendations are implemented effectively and safely and (b) that the interventions are directly addressing the child's needs and supporting her performance across environments.

In Chapter 4, we will start by a review of evidence-based interventions for ASD and then present programs that have proven effective for students with sensory issues.

INTERVENTIONS FOR SENSORY ISSUES

As mentioned, many children and youth with high-functioning autism spectrum disorders (HF-ASD) exhibit a variety of behaviors in school, home, and community that interfere with their ability to meet the demands of school as well as make and keep friends. Understanding that behaviors may have underlying sensory components helps guide us in interpreting and planning strategies to support these children across settings.

We would not presume that ALL behaviors exhibited by individuals with HF-ASD have an underlying sensory cause, but given that up to 95% of these individuals experience sensory issues (Baker, Lane, Angley, & Young, 2008; Baranek et al., 2006; Dunn, Myles & Orr, 2002; Tomchek & Dunn, 2007), it is extremely important to include a sensory approach.

This chapter starts out with a brief overview of the research on evidence-based practices followed by some programs that address sensory issues. Based on the premise that all behaviors have a purpose, the chapter then goes on to focus on intervention strategies that address behaviors often seen in children with HF-ASD that may have a sensory basis.

Evidence-Based Practices and Sensory Interventions

In recent years, emphasis has been placed on identifying evidence-based practices (EBP) for all learners, including those on the autism spectrum. To date, five reports have been have been published on this topic, by the National Autism Center (NAC 2009), National Professional Development Center on Autism (NPDC on ASD, 2009), Agency for Healthcare Research and Policy

(AHRQ, 2011), Centers for Medicaid and Medicare Services (CMS, 2010), and the Texas Statewide Leadership for Autism Training (2011).

In order to determine whether studies on interventions were scientifically rigorous, the first report, from the NPDC on ASD (2009), used the following criteria for articles on interventions used with individuals with ASD (excluding intervention packages): (a) at least two experimental or quasi-experimental group design studies carried out by independent investigators, (b) at least five single-case design studies from at least three independent investigators, or (c) a combination of at least one experimental/quasi-experimental study and three single-case design studies from independent investigators.

The authors of the second report (NAC, 2009) developed a Scientific Merit Rating Scale (SMRS) that analyzed within an article (a) research design, (b) measurement of the dependent variable, (c) measurement of the independent variable or procedural fidelity, (d) participant ascertainment, and (e) generalization. Each of these elements was subsequently rated on a 5-point Likert scale with scores of 3, 4, or 5 indicating scientific rigor.

The third report, commissioned by the Centers for Medicare and Medicaid Services (CMS, 2010), sought to determine scientific evidence of the efficacy, effectiveness, safety, and availability of ASD-related psychosocial services and supports for children, transitioning youth, and adults with ASD. Articles on interventions were classified as evidence based using the criteria adopted by the NPDC on ASD and the categories identified by the NAC.

The fourth report, written for AHRQ (2011) used the following criteria: (a) study design that included randomized controlled trials (RCT), prospective and retrospective studies, non-RCT, case-control studies and case series; (b) sample sizes greater than 10; (c) rigorous diagnostic approach; (c) participant ascertainment; (d) treatment fully described with fidelity; and (e) valid and reliable outcome measures. Studies were rated as good, fair, or poor by a technical expert panel (TEP).

The final report, commissioned by the Texas Statewide Leadership for Autism Training (2011), used the following definition of EBP, "The best measure of effectiveness of an intervention is whether it is effective for a particular individual. It is of utmost importance to collect and analyze data when using interventions with a student with autism. If an intervention results in positive change for a particular student and you, as an educational professional, have data to support that, then the intervention is evidence-based for that student" (para 6).[1]

---

1 Information on where to find these reports is found in the References section.

Sensory Interventions

Sensory interventions were not directly identified as evidence based in the afore-mentioned reports. However, one category of interventions, antecedent-based interventions – under which sensory interventions are classified – was identified by three of the reports. Antecedent-based interventions are described as, "Modifications of events that typically precede the occurrence of a target behavior. These alterations are made to increase the likelihood of success or reduce the likelihood of problems" … and … "Include (a) using highly preferred activities/items to increase interest level, (b) changing schedule/routine, (c) implementing preactivity interventions, (d) offering choices, (e) altering the manner in which instruction is provided, and (f) enriching the environment for access to sensory stimuli that serve the same function as the interfering behavior" (Smith, Myles, Aspy, Grossman, & Henry, 2010, p. 5) [underlines are for emphasis]. This clearly refers to and applies to sensory interventions.

Further, three randomized controlled trials were conducted on sensory interventions. All showed significant changes in the group that received sensory interventions compared to the control group:

- Fazlioglu, Y., & Baran, G. (2008). A sensory integration therapy program on sensory problems for children with autism. *Perceptual Motor Skills, 106*(2), 415-422.

- Pfeiffer, B., Koenig, K., Kinnealey, M., Sheppard, M., & Henderson, L. (2011). Effectiveness of sensory integration interventions in children with autism spectrum disorders: A pilot study. *American Journal of Occupational Therapy, 65*, 76-85.

- Smith, S. A., Press, B., Koenig, K. P., & Kinnealey, M. (2005). Effects of sensory integration intervention on self-stimulating and self-injurious behaviors. *American Journal of Occupational Therapy, 59*, 418-425.

How do these studies fit within the EBP reports? The NAC included reports published through fall 2007. Thus, two of the three studies were not evaluated. But these studies may meet the criteria established by CMS and NPDC: at least two experimental or quasi-experimental group design studies carried out by independent investigators. The AHRQ report (a) rated the Fazlioğlu and Baran (2008) study as "fair"; (b) did not evaluate the Pfeiffer et al. (2011) study, presumably due to the publication date; and (c) did not evaluate the Smith et al. (2005) because it did not meet the inclusion criteria of a sample size of more than 10 in each group.

Selected Publications and Programs That Address the Sensory and Regulation Needs of Children and Youth With HF-ASD

Several programs appear effective in meeting the sensory needs of children and youth with HF-ASD. We have not attempted to provide a comprehensive list but have highlighted some of the programs with which we have experienced success in working with individuals with HF-ASD. These include the following.

- **A Buffet of Sensory Interventions: Solutions for Middle and High School Students (Culp, 2011).** This practical resource focuses on middle and high school students, whose sensory and regulation needs are often overlooked. The author emphasizes the importance of fostering independence, self-advocacy, and self-regulation as a way for teens with ASD to take ownership of their sensory needs as they transition into adulthood.

- **The ECLIPSE Model: Teaching Self-Regulation, Executive Function, Attribution, and Sensory Awareness to Students With Asperger Syndrome, High-functioning Autism, and Related Disorders (Moyer & NHS, 2009).** This model targets the skills needed to improve social competence, such as executive functioning, theory of mind, causal attribution, processing speed, sensory regulation, and working memory. Without effective use of these skills on a regular basis, development of other areas of functioning – academic, adaptive, social and vocational skills – is inhibited. The ECLIPSE Model directly addresses four critical challenge areas that are not typically covered by other curricula: self-regulation, executive function, attribution retraining, and sensory awareness.

- **The Incredible 5-Point Scale (rev. ed.; Buron & Curtis 2012).** This resource shows how the use of a simple 5-point scale can help students understand and regulate their behavior. The book shows how to break down a given behavior and, with the student's active participation, develop a scale that identifies the problem and suggests alternative, positive behaviors at each level of the scale.

- **Learn to Move, Move to Learn "Family" (Brack, 2004, 2005, 2009).** Two books follow a sensory integrated developmental sequence of activities related to the theme. For maximum flexibility, suggestions for adaptation and modification for individual students are included, along with instructions for how to develop additional lessons. A companion DVD gives a first-hand view of real children engaged in a dinosaur theme-based sensorimotor lesson and thus sparks ideas for other similar activities. In addition, a CD of 25 songs teaches children to regulate their sensory system.

• **My Sensory Book: Working Together to Explore Sensory Issues and the Big Feelings They Can Cause: A Workbook for Parents, Professionals, and Children (Kerstein, 2008).** This interactive workbook enables children to develop a better understanding of their sensory systems by helping their parents and teachers create an individualized sensory profile. Through numerous strategies broken down by the different sensory systems, children can learn to cope more effectively with the world around them.

• **Hygiene and Related Behaviors for Children and Adolescents With Autism Spectrum and Related Disorders: A Fun Curriculum With a Focus on Social Understanding (Mahler, 2009).** This curriculum teaches important hygiene skills using a fun approach that targets the core characteristics, including sensory needs, and learning styles of children and adolescents on the spectrum. Ranging from basic daily hygiene to picking, using public restrooms, and burping and farting, topics focus on healthy and socially acceptable behaviors.

• **Sensory Processing Disorder: Simulations and Solutions for Parents, Teachers, and Therapists DVD and Kit (Brack, 2006).** This DVD allows viewers to experience what it feels like to have sensory challenges. By engaging in simulated exercises for a variety of sensory processing difficulties, viewers will learn not only basic information about sensory systems, but also how to deal with sensory challenges both at home and at school.

• **Building Bridges Through Sensory Integration (Yack, Sutton, & Aquilla, 2nd ed., 2003).** Designed to help educators and parents develop insight into the sensory needs of children, this books specifically focuses on children who have been diagnosed with autism and other related exceptionalities. Within this resource, checklists help the reader identify children's difficulties in (a) general self-care, (b) dressing, (c) eating, (d) school/work, (e) play, and (f) social skills. In addition, activities are included that address environmental and behavioral accommodations.

- **How Does Your Engine Run?: A Leader's Guide to the Alert Program for Self-Regulation (Williams & Shellenberger, 1996).** Intended for use by occupational therapists in conjunction with educators and parents, this program helps children recognize their sensory needs. In addition, children and youth learn to recognize their level of alertness or arousal and to change that level as necessary to meet academic or social demands.

- **The Tool Chest for Teachers, Parents, and Students (Henry Occupational Therapy Services, 1998).** This resource provides 26 activities to assist educators and parents in helping children meet their sensory needs. This self-guided handbook discusses how to identify what a behavior may be communicating and how to develop strategies that will prevent behavior problems from occurring. Each activity outlines its benefits, where to begin, strategy instructions, additional projects, and supplies needed. The text is supplemented by two videos.

In addition, materials have been published that address the often sensory-related regulation challenges of individuals with HF-ASD. These include:

- **Outsmarting Explosive Behavior: A Visual System of Support and Intervention for Individuals With Autism Spectrum Disorders (Endow, 2009).** This program is designed to help decrease – and in some cases eliminate – explosive behavior in children with HF-ASD. This visual program is laid out as a fold-out poster that can be individualized for each user. Four train cars represent the four stages of explosive behavior. The program makes it easy to help learners identify their current state and take steps to decrease the chances of a meltdown.

- **Asperger Syndrome and Difficult Moments: Practical Solutions for Tantrums, Rage, and Meltdowns, (2nd ed; Myles & Southwick, 2005).** This book offers solutions to minimize and circumvent the often frightening circumstances that surround the rage cycle – not only for the child with HF-ASD but others in the environment as well. This detailed book takes the reader through the stages of the rage cycle, emphasizing the importance of regulation, understanding the sensory environment, and teachable moments.

Two comprehensive planning models – the Ziggurat Model and the Comprehensive Autism Planning System – embed sensory interventions into assessment and programming for individuals on the spectrum.

- **Designing Comprehensive Interventions for High-Functioning Individuals With Autism Spectrum Disorders: The Ziggurat Model – Release 2.0. (Aspy & Grossman, 2011).** The Ziggurat Model begins with an assessment of underlying needs and characteristics. To that end, the model includes the Underlying Characteristics Checklist (UCC) that provides a snapshot of how ASD is expressed for an individual. Three forms of this instrument exist – the UCC-HF for individuals with HF-ASD, the UCC-CL for individuals with a classic presentation of autism, and the UCC-EI for infants and toddlers. The Intervention Ziggurat contains five levels derived from research on ASD (see Table 4.1). Interventions at each level are selected to match the student's true needs (identified with the UCC) to ensure that "the autism" is addressed. Thus, interventions are meaningful – meeting underlying needs instead of masking them.

Table 4.1
Components of the Intervention Ziggurat

Components	Brief Overview
Sensory Differences and Biological Needs	The impact of each of the seven sensory systems on the individual with ASD is considered in this section of the Ziggurat. In addition, biological considerations, such as medication, allergies, and sleep needs, are taken into consideration.
Reinforcement	Reinforcement, an essential component of student learning, is integrated into the Ziggurat framework. Student preferences, including special interests, support the acquisition and maintenance of skills.
Structure and Visual/Tactile Support	These supports are integral to creating a learning environment that is predictable and rich in language. This Ziggurat level addresses classroom layout, home base, visual schedules, choice boards, boundary markers, communication systems, learning style, modes of expressing and receiving language and academic/pre-academic modifications.
Task Demands	An often overlooked instructional component, task demand interventions are designed to ensure that students are not required to participate in activities or to complete assignments that exceed their abilities. A reduction of demands and the addition of supports is required to facilitate success.
Skills to Teach	Finally, this Ziggurat area includes the skills, tasks, and/or behaviors on which the student requires direct instruction in order to experience success.

- **The Comprehensive Autism Planning System (CAPS) for Individuals With Autism Spectrum Disorders and Related Disabilities: Integrating Evidence-Based Practices Throughout the Student's Day (rev. ed.; Henry & Myles, 2013).** CAPS is designed to provide an overview of a student's daily schedule by time and activity as well as the supports that are needed during each period. Following the development of the student's IEP, all educational professionals who work with the student develop the CAPS. The CAPS allows professionals and parents to answer the all-important question: What supports does the student need for each activity? The CAPS is a list of a student's daily tasks and activities, the times they occur, along with the delineation of supports needed for student success. In addition, the CAPS includes space for making notations about data collection and how skills are to be generalized to others settings. CAPS consists of the following components developed from evidence-based best practices for students with ASD: (a) time, (b) activity, (c) targeted skills to teach, (d) structure/modifications, (e) reinforcement, (f) sensory strategies, (g) communication/social skills, (h) data collection, and (i) generalization plan.

Children's books are helpful in helping learners on the spectrum understand their sensory and regulation challenges. Examples of such books include:

- **Arnie and His School Tools: Simple Sensory Solutions That Build Success (Veenendall, 2010).** This illustrated book centers around an exuberant little boy who had difficulty paying attention in class and doing his schoolwork until he was equipped with tools that helped accommodate his sensory needs. Resources for adults are provided at the end of the book, including definitions, suggested discussion questions, and lists of related books and web sites.

- **The Chameleon Kid: Controlling Meltdown Before He Controls You (Larson, 2008).** Much like the chameleon, the child with HF-ASD can adapt to his surroundings by altering his behavior in dealing with the emotions that precede a meltdown. By practicing the techniques in *The Chameleon Kid*, children can learn to eliminate Meltdown, depicted as a monster, or at least reduce its hold on him. The dramatic and colorful page spreads literally show readers in front of their own eyes how the Chameleon Kid reduces Meltdown in size and power by using the strategies presented in the book.

- **A "5" Could Make Me Lose Control! An Activity-Based Method for Evaluating and Supporting Highly Anxious Students (Buron, 2007).** This hands-on activity helps students who are highly anxious cope with their stress by classifying social, sensory and emotional information and analyzing how best to act.

- **When My Worries Get Too Big! A Relaxation Book for Children Who Live With Anxiety – Revised and Expanded Edition (Buron, 2013).** This book allows young children to explore their own feelings when they react to events in their daily lives and to participate in developing their own self-calming strategies. Teaching activities provide a practical springboard for discussion and exploration.

- **The Way to A: Empowering Children With Autism Spectrum and Other Neurological Disorders to Monitor and Replace Aggression and Tantrum Behavior (Manasco, 2006).** This book presents a simple, logical, and systematic strategy that clarifies and sequentially teaches the child how to regulate his behavior by engaging in forethought and self-analysis before acting out. What sets this strategy apart is that it then goes on to give the child a personal and concrete incentive to use the alternative behavior.

- **Why Does Izzy Cover Her Ears? Dealing With Sensory Overload (Veenendall, 2009).** Izzy is a feisty first grader whose behavior is often misunderstood as she tries to cope with sensory overload in her new surroundings. The book creates an environment that is accepting of students with sensory and regulation difficulties. Resources for adults at the end of the book include definitions of sensory processing and sensory modulation disorder, suggested discussion questions and lists of related books and web sites.

Incidents, Interpretations, and Interventions

In addition to the aforementioned programs and books used to systematically address sensory issues, it is sometimes necessary to act "on the spot" and implement sensory-based strategies that address the exact cause of the specific sensory issue observed. Table 4.2 provides many examples of this process. It is organized into three columns:

- incident – description of the behavior you may see

- interpretation – possible sensory-based reason(s) why the behavior occurs

- intervention – sensory-based strategies and supports

Many of the supports or interventions are easy to implement both at school and at home. It is best for parents and professionals to work together as a team to pinpoint the behavior a child exhibits (incident), its cause (interpretation), and practical solutions (intervention). An occupational therapist or someone trained in sensory integration can be a particularly valuable multidisciplinary team member.

Table 4.2

Incidents, Interpretations, and Interventions

Incident	Interpretation	Intervention
ACCIDENT PRONE		
Has trouble pouring and carrying without spilling	• Has trouble with motor planning related to successfully completing task. • May require additional proprioceptive input to judge body movements and adjustments needed.	• Increase the weight of the container while decreasing the amount of liquid in it. • Use dishes that are heavier to carry. • Have the child carry items to the table, using containers that will not spill on the way to the table. • Fill cups or bowls only partially. • Please consult with an OT.
Is clumsy/accident prone; bumps into things and breaks things often.	• Difficulty judging body positioning in relation to objects in the environment.	• Provide proprioceptive input using weighted vest, or ankle or wrist weights. • Teach the child to visually monitor movements in the environment.
Seems impulsive or hurries through things, including being unaware of safety issues.	• May have difficulty planning and including all steps in the appropriate order of performance. • May be avoiding contact with materials or activities that are perceived as unpleasant.	• Break the activity into steps and ask the child to perform one step at a time, completing each step before moving on. • Have someone model the activity first. • Use a visual for each step. • Reinforce completion of each step instead of just the final project. • Consider tactile sensitivity or avoidance and provide an alternate material with less threatening sensory features (i.e., use a cotton swab to glue on small pieces of the art activity instead of getting glue on fingers). • Consider a cooperative assignment where different steps can be distributed among students.

Table 4.2 (continued)

Incident	Interpretation	Intervention
ATTENTION		
Doesn't seem to understand body language or facial expressions.	• May be uncomfortable directing visual attention to body parts, body movements, or the faces of others. • May have difficulty processing the many changes in body movements and facial expressions. • May have problems distinguishing meaningful visual information from competing visual background detail. • Awareness of other individuals in the surrounding environment may be limited by intense preoccupation or focus. • Maintaining a distance from others to avoid physical touch could limit ability to perceive body language and facial expressions. • May be reliant on auditory information to guide actions.	• Provide auditory cue to direct attention. • Use an inflatable disc or camping pillow during times when concentration is needed. • Teach the meanings of facial expressions, specific body postures and gestures. • Whenever possible, eliminate some of the background distractors that may be present in the environment. • Respect the individual's need for distance to avoid physical touch. Verbally reassure her. Request that she watch you for specific cues. • Accompany facial expressions, gestures and body language with spoken language. • Be aware of the use of unspoken cues when delivering instruction. • Try to use as few sensory modalities at a time as possible.
Has problems making eye contact with others.	• Peripheral visual information may be more comfortable or useful than central vision. • May be difficult to "look" and "listen" at the same time. • May lack confidence about abilities. • Movement activities may be more comfortable or successful if the child is able to fix visual gaze on something besides another person.	• Consider decreasing expectation of "eye contact" in some situations and contexts. • Position in "line of sight" without getting too close. • Provide minimal auditory or slight tactile cue to encourage visual attention. • Incorporate activities that facilitate looking through labeling, turn taking and obtaining information and objects from others. Example: Have the child swing while asking him to label items being shown to him, held near the adult's face. • Break down tasks to smaller steps where success will be more readily achieved. • Provide imitation opportunities and activities for child to repeat a modeled behavior or action.

Table 4.2 (continued)

Incident	Interpretation	Intervention
ATTENTION (continued)		
Stares intensely at people	• Has difficulty knowing which stimuli to attend to. • May need additional time to process information from his environment. • Visual acuity may be less than optimal. • Has a low tolerance for movement, subsequently limiting head movements. • Auditory comprehension problems may cause child to seek more intense visual information to compensate. • May be visually fixating on a target not related to the task as a way to aid in concentration or to prevent sensory overload.	• Develop auditory or visual cues that the child can use to help him know what to attend to. • Provide direct instruction on how to shift attention. Use imitation games (i.e., "Simon Says") to reinforce the skill. • Provide a written script that tells the student how to shift attention. • Provide a social narrative that discusses how others feel when people stare at them.
BEHAVIOR IN GROUPS		
Doesn't seem to understand body language or facial expressions.	• May be uncomfortable directing visual attention to body parts, body movements, or the faces of others. • May have difficulty processing the many changes in body movements and facial expressions. • May have problems distinguishing meaningful visual information from competing visual background detail. • Awareness of other individuals in the surrounding environment may be limited by intense preoccupation or focus. • Maintaining a distance from others to avoid physical touch could limit ability to perceive body language and facial expressions. • May be reliant on auditory information to guide actions.	• Provide auditory cue to direct attention. • Use a Disc 'O' Sit™ or camping pillow during times when concentration is needed. • Teach the meanings of facial expressions, specific body postures, and gestures. • Whenever possible, eliminate some of the background distractors that may be present in the environment. • Respect the individual's need for distance to avoid physical touch. • Verbally reassure her. Request that she watch you for specific cues. • Accompany facial expressions, gestures, and body language with spoken language. • Be aware of the use of unspoken cues when delivering instruction. • Try to use as few sensory modalities at a time as possible.

Table 4.2 (continued)

Incident	Interpretation	Intervention
BEHAVIOR IN GROUPS (continued)		
Has difficulty keeping hands and feet to self when sitting in groups.	• Craves tactile input. • Doesn't understand about personal boundaries. • May learn by handling or manipulating objects.	• Provide visual or physical boundaries for sitting such as tape boundaries, carpet squares, placemats, inflatable disc, or camping pillow. • Provide a "fidget item" such as a Koosh Ball™ or Tangle™. Often fidget items can be academically related, such as holding a play cow when studying farm animals or grasping a squeeze/stress ball that looks like a planet when studying the solar system. • If the reaction occurs during a floor-based activity, have child lie on her stomach, propping her head on her elbows. • Have child hold or squeeze a large pillow held in lap.
Has difficulty regulating reactions in the lunchroom, including going into a tantrum, screaming, or refusing to cooperate.	• Situations that have loud echoes, noise, movement, and strong scents can be stressful.	• Allow the child to go to the cafeteria early. • Allow the child to eat in the classroom or other nonstimulating environment. • Decrease time in the lunchroom. • Assist the child in setting up for the meal (opening milk, condiments, helping to select food).
Has problems making eye contact with others.	• Peripheral visual information may be more comfortable or useful than central vision. • May be difficult to "look" and "listen" at the same time. • May lack confidence in abilities. • Movement activities may be more comfortable or successful if the child is able to fix visual gaze on something besides another person.	• Consider decreasing expectation of "eye contact" in some situations and contexts. • Position in "line of sight" without getting too close. • Provide minimal auditory or slight tactile cue to encourage visual attention. • Incorporate activities that facilitate looking through labeling, turn taking, and obtaining information and objects from others. Example: Have the child swing while asking him to label items being shown to him, held near the adult's face. • Break down tasks to smaller steps where success will be more readily achieved. • Provide imitation opportunities and activities for child to repeat a modeled behavior or action.
Leans on peers while in line, sitting in groups, or sitting at table.	• May have poor postural control. • May require proprioceptive or vestibular input; his central nervous system may need "waking up."	• Provide opportunities for large-motor activities such as jumping, pulling and pushing prior to these activities. • Allow the child to stand during activities. • Provide the child legitimate opportunities to move, such as sharpening pencils or throwing away trash. • Place rubberized shelf-lining or Dycem™ on the seat of the chair. • Place a tennis ball on two chair legs (diagonal). This allows for continual small movements.

Table 4.2 (continued)

Incident	Interpretation	Intervention
BEHAVIOR IN GROUPS (continued)		
Steps on peers' heels/feet when walking, misses the chair when attempting to sit down, or sits on peers when group is sitting on the floor.	• Poor awareness. • Difficulty planning motor actions. • May have poor proprioceptive processing.	• At the preschool or early elementary level, consider having the child hop, skip, do jumping jacks, bend down and touch toes half way down the hall (depending on motor planning ability). These activities may also be effective if done within the classroom just before walking down the hall. • Consider placing the student at the front or back of the line. • Ensure appropriate amount of spacing between students in line. • Instruct the child to carry her books against her body with hands touching opposite elbows.
DRESSING/CLOTHES		
Always looks unkempt/sloppy.	• Has decreased body awareness or has difficulty "feeling" that his clothes are not on straight.	• Create a visual schedule for getting ready. • Have the child wear clothing that is "snug" to provide an increased awareness. • Teach the child a sequential strategy for evaluating appearance (i.e., when leaving for the bus stop, check mirror for combed hair, no toothpaste on mouth, shirt buttoned correctly, pants zipped, shoes tied).
Can't stand sand in shoes or bumps of seams in socks.	• Feel of sand or seams is extremely uncomfortable.	• Turn socks inside out so the seam is on the outside. • Try different socks where the seams are not as prominent. • Be aware of the type of shoes the child is wearing. • Select shoes for comfort, not style.
Dislikes certain clothes.	• Certain textures or materials may be more irritating than others. • Characteristics of specific items may be irritating and uncomfortable for the child such as sleeve length or certain forms of waistbands. Some dislike the sound of nylon or corduroy pants when walking.	• Respect the child's desire for certain textures when appropriate. • Rub lotion on the child. • Massage the child with a vigorous towel rub to increase tolerance to certain textures of clothing items and then introduce a new item or texture. • Remove clothing tags that may cause irritation. • Use one detergent consistently. • Consider a fragrance-free detergent.

Table 4.2 *(continued)*

Incident	Interpretation	Intervention
DRESSING/CLOTHES *(continued)*		
Refuses to go barefoot, especially in grass.	• Feet may be very sensitive.	• Try rubbing the child's feet with a cloth or towel first. • Introduce new textures to the child's feet such as sand, beans, rice, bubble wrap, or Contact Paper™. Offer but do not force these activities. • Provide the child with socks that have a new "feel."
Trouble dressing, especially clothes with fasteners.	• Has difficulty with fine-motor skills. • May have weak hand muscles.	• Have the child work with Velcro fasteners. • Begin with larger fasteners or buttons. Once these have been mastered, move to smaller fasteners or buttons. • Buy clothes that have few or no fasteners. • Tell the child to look as she fastens. • Instruct the child to start with the bottom fastener, snap, or button. • Use activities to increase hand strength (i.e., using therapy putty, clay or Playdoh™ with small objects hidden within it. Have the child pull the therapy putty apart to look for the items.
Wears clothing inappropriate for the situation – no boots or coat in snow.	• Texture and style of clothing may be irritating.	• Ensure that clothes apply the appropriate pressure and are of a texture that is comfortable to the child. • Make allowances for individual preferences, when appropriate. • Gradually introduce new clothes. For example, for younger children introduce an item that a favorite doll can wear. For older children, introduce a new item that contains a desired logo or television character.
EATING/CHEWING		
Chews on clothing, pens, pencils.	• May find this calming. • May be seeking proprioceptive input. • May like the tactile input of the item.	• Allow the child to chew on gum, gummy worms (chill to harden), jujubes, hard candy, coffee stirrers, latex-free tubing, straws, or have snacks that are crunchy or chewy. • Allow the child to chew on clothes if it does not cause harm. • Provide a water bottle with a sturdy straw that the child can drink from. • Consider alternatives with a strong oral emphasis.
Is easily distracted/ nauseated by certain smells.	• May be oversensitive to certain smells and become very irritated when exposed to them.	• Use unscented detergents or shampoos. • Refrain from wearing perfumes or aftershave lotions that are irritating to the child. • Make the environment as fragrance-free as possible.

Table 4.2 (continued)

Incident	Interpretation	Intervention
EATING/CHEWING (continued)		
Is easily distracted/nauseated by certain tastes.	• May be very sensitive to certain textures or tastes of foods.	• Respect individual differences if nutrition is not compromised. • Change one characteristic of food at a time. If the child likes fruit, dehydrate the fruit to introduce a new texture. Mix two preferred fruits. • Introduce very small bites or portions.
Messy eater; prefers to use fingers rather than utensils to eat.	• May be unable to "feel" the sensation around the mouth area. • Dislikes the feel of the utensils in his mouth or hands. • May have poor fine-motor skills.	• Massage lightly around the child's mouth using different materials and textures such as washcloths, soft-bristled toothbrush, or mini-vibrating toothbrush. • Encourage activities that involve the mouth (i.e., whistles, bubble wands, kazoos).
Won't eat certain foods.	• Texture of the food may not be pleasant. • May be sensitive to the temperature of the food items. • May be oversensitive to certain tastes.	• Allow the child to choose foods as long as nutrition is not compromised. • Apply deep pressure to teeth and gums using a hard, yet pliable item. For example, chewing on rubber tubing or a straw may help the child. • Introduce new foods by expanding one sensory characteristic at a time. For example, if the child eats yogurt, introduce corn flakes, oat flakes, or grape nuts into the yogurt to provide texture.
EMOTIONS/FEELINGS/RELATIONSHIPS		
Appears to like father's touch better than mother's.	• Mother's touch may be too light. • May not anticipate mother's touch because mother walks up quietly behind the child. Father's touch may be anticipated because the child may hear father coming or father may always approach head-on.	• Make the child aware that touch is coming. • Allow the child to initiate the touch.
Dislikes being hugged or kissed, but is okay when he initiates.	• Touch may be uncomfortable if unexpected.	• When appropriate, allow the child to determine when he will hug or kiss. • Enlighten family members or friends about the child's preferences to avoid uncomfortable and embarrassing situations. • Let the child know before a hug or kiss takes place.

Table 4.2 (continued)

Incident	Interpretation	Intervention
EMOTIONS/FEELINGS/RELATIONSHIPS (continued)		
Has difficulty making friends.	• Poor motor planning skills impact success at group activities and games. • Decreased (hyposensitivity) awareness of food and materials on face and hands limits social acceptance. • Hypersensitivity to incidental or unplanned touch may result in reactionary behaviors not understood by others. • May fail to observe and comprehend the meaning of gestures and facial expressions. • Self-talk and other anxiety-reducing behaviors may interfere with conversational skills. • Restricted interest or preoccupation with objects or activities may decrease sensory availability for other people and things in the environment, impacting opportunities for spontaneous play. • Unpredictable emotional reactions may impact the child's ability to form friendships.	• Establish a structured recess activity with preassigned roles that can be practiced in isolation. • Teach a self-care routine such as using a napkin after every 3 bites or handwashing following each recess. • Practice a socially acceptable "script" that could be expressed by the child when unexpectedly bumped. • Teach the child how to approach an individual or group as well as the skills needed to interact with peers. • Provide direct instruction for common gestures and expressions with opportunities to practice observation skills in a non-threatening situation. • Provide a hand fidget that can be discreetly manipulated, leaving visual attention available. • Develop a "Circle of Friends," "Lunch Bunch," or "Recess Buddies" for the child. • Develop an integrated play group that involves the child and typical peers that will include various sensory motor activities.
Is sensitive to criticism.	• May have poor self-concept about abilities based on motor planning difficulties that result in uncoordinated movements. • Overconfidence may be a defense mechanism for coping with motor planning difficulties. • May be reacting to sensory characteristics of the person providing the criticism (i.e., voice quality, volume, pitch) rather than the criticism itself. • Anxiety about skills or performance affects ability to generate ideas or problem-solve.	• Deliver feedback in a positive manner at a time when the child is emotionally available. • Consider providing feedback visually through cartooning, social stories, or social autopsy. • Provide opportunities for the child to identify his strengths and discuss characteristics that can be a concern. • Present potentially difficult tasks with models, written or pictorial directions, and structure. • Model how to react to criticism. • Teach the child a strategy of how to respond to criticism.

Table 4.2 (continued)

Incident	Interpretation	Intervention
GROOMING		
Dislikes having face or hair washed.	• Light touch may be painful or annoying.	• Allow the child to wash her own hair. The response is often less defensive if the child regulates the touching herself. • Use firm pressure. Deep pressure does not elicit as strong an emotional response. • Let the child know she is going to be touched before it occurs.
Dislikes toothbrushing.	• Toothbrush may be too big or the bristles too hard. • Taste or texture of the toothpaste may be irritating to the child's nervous system.	• Consider a smaller toothbrush with softer bristles or a toothbrush that vibrates. • If possible, let the child control his own toothbrush. That way, he can control the amount of pressure that is comfortable to tolerate. • Select toothpaste that tastes good to the child. • Monitor the amount of toothpaste on the toothbrush. • Consider dipping the damp toothbrush into the toothpaste instead of squeezing a "blob" on it.
Does not like having hair cut.	• May be sensitive to the movement and height or overall size of the barber chair. • Head movement required to lie back in sink may be unpleasant. • Errant spray from sink nozzle or spray bottle may be annoying. • Noise and vibration of clippers or scissors may be unsettling. • Visual and tactile sensitivity may be triggered by close proximity of barber. • Sensation around neck and noise of vinyl drape may be uncomfortable. • Has trouble with feel of stray, cut hair on neck and clothes following haircut.	• Provide a visual support that outlines the steps of getting a hair cut. • For the younger child, play-act giving a doll or stuffed animal a pretend haircut, verbally elaborating on the sensory aspects that are a part of the process. • Prepare child with verbal instruction such as "I'm going to raise the chair now." • Provide the opportunity for the child to make choices about the process. • Invite the child to participate in the process — "Do you want to spray your own hair?" • Cut hair in a chair with surrounding support. Place pillows under and around child. • Provide favorable music, using earbuds to listen if needed. • Apply deep pressure to the child's head before beginning the hair cut. This can be done directly using the fingertips or a towel may be used to rub the head. • Allow the child to manipulate a fidget or hold a small vibrator in his hands while his hair is being cut. Give the child a Koosh™ ball, Theraputty™, or some sort of character with moveable body parts to play with during the hair cut. • Provide an alternative to the standard drape like a towel. • Bring fresh clothing for child to change into following the haircut. • Consider providing a preferred activity following the hair cut.

Table 4.2 *(continued)*

Incident	Interpretation	Intervention
GROOMING *(continued)*		
Does not like having nails cut.	• The actual cutting of the nail may be painful or uncomfortable for the child. • Having another person hold the child's finger may be uncomfortable for the child. • Fear of cutting too close to the quick or cutting skin may be anxiety-provoking.	• Rub the child's hands with lotion using deep pressure before beginning to cut the nails. • Try cuticle scissors as they may be more tolerable than larger fingernail clippers. • Use an emery board in lieu of clipping nails to keep at a manageable length. • Try cutting the child's nails while he is interested in or distracted by something else, maybe even sleeping. • Cut nails as part of the bathing routine following playtime when the nail is softer and more pliable. • Break the task into smaller increments such as two fingers at a time over a period of time. • Have the child place fingers over a table or counter edge pressing down to provide deep pressure to the fingertip but leaving nail edge exposed for clipping. • Use a social narrative to describe the steps of nail clipping and the hygiene and social benefits of well-groomed nails.
MOVEMENT		
Has difficulty transitioning in hallways. (Note: Response may depend on amount of activity in the hallway.)	• May be touched unexpectedly by somebody. The touch may be misinterpreted as a hit, causing a defensive response. • Noise in the hall may be too loud. • Visual activity may be disorienting.	• Allow the child to be first or last in line. • Allow the child to leave class 5 minutes early. • Have the child carry something heavy to provide proprioceptive input. • Create a map that provides a visual plan or route between locations. • Have the child hold the door open for the rest of the class by leaning her back into the door. This extra input may help her tolerate the subsequent sensory input of the hall. • Consider preferential placement of locker (at the end of the row) to decrease opportunities for unintentional physical contact with other students.
Prefers only to engage in sedentary activities (i.e., television, computer, video games).	• Limiting actions may be a way to avoid activities that present unpleasant sensations and unpredictable movements. • May have poor self-concept about abilities based on motor planning difficulties that result in uncoordinated movements. • Anxiety about skills or performance affects his ability to generate ideas or problem-solve.	• Embed physical movement into routine activities such as making the bed, emptying the trash, pushing the book cart, etc. • Incorporate movement into the child's sedentary activity. For example, to play a video game, the child must first walk up a flight of stairs or get the video game from the highest shelf. • Add music to the task providing a structured starting and stopping point. • Utilize the child's area of interest to elaborate on the activity. • Provide a visual support that demonstrates the steps of a nonsedentary activity.

Table 4.2 (continued)

Incident	Interpretation	Intervention
MOVEMENT *(continued)*		
Steps on peers' heels/feet when talking, misses the chair when attempting to sit down, or sits on peers when group is sitting on the floor.	• Poor awareness. • Difficulty planning motor actions.	• At the preschool or early elementary level, consider having the child hop, skip, do jumping jacks, bend down and touch toes half way down the hall (depending on motor planning ability). These activities may also be effective if done within the classroom just before walking down the hall. • Consider placing the student at the front or back of the line. • Ensure appropriate amount of spacing between students in line. • Instruct the child to carry her books against her body with hands touching opposite elbows. • Teach the child a song that she can sing to herself while walking down the hall (*Personal Space Invaders*, Lyons, 1997).
NOISE/SOUND		
Does not notice sounds in the environment.	• Has a difficult time knowing which sounds to attend to. • May be so focused on what he is doing that the sound does not register. • May have difficulty perceiving specific pitches or frequencies.	• Plan activities that will help teach the child to attend to various sounds. Play games using various sounds found in the environment like an auditory bingo game. • Utilize a visual or tactile cue to gain the child's attention.
Does not respond when name is called.	• May be so focused on what she is doing that the sound does not register. • May have difficulty perceiving specific pitches or frequencies.	• Teach the child to attend to his name by using games that involve saying his name and then reinforcing him for responding. • Develop visual cues or signals to gain the child's attention. • Vary the intonation or add melody, using a "sing-song" manner. • Pair a novel auditory cue with name such as clicking fingers or clapping hands.
Easily distracted by and fearful of loud noise.	• May be hypersensitive to noises, especially when not prepared for them. • May have difficulty determining which noises or tones to attend to in the environment and which to disregard.	• Use soft talking or singing to help the child know what to attend to. • Use soft background noise for calming. • In situations or places where the child experiences a lot of loud noises, have the child wear headphones or earplugs to buffer some of the noise. • Whenever possible, alert or prepare the child before the offending noise occurs. • Avoid using appliances or equipment at times when you would like the child to maintain his focus.

Table 4.2 *(continued)*

Incident	Interpretation	Intervention
NOISE/SOUND *(continued)*		
Has difficulty processing sounds.	• When exposed to several sounds at the same time, it may be difficult for the child to know which sounds to attend to and when to attend to them.	• Get the child's attention first. Give directions slowly, allowing time for the child to process in between each step. • After giving directions, ask the child to repeat what was said to check for accuracy. • Use body gestures and/or visual supports along with the verbal directions. • Make sure that quiet occurs before directions are given. • Teach a cue to use when the child needs to attend (i.e., hand signal, touch on the shoulder).
Hums constantly.	• May be overstimulated by classroom noise. The humming may block out noises that cause anxiety. • Seeks auditory or tactile input.	• If the noise or activity level is a concern, move the child away from the source of noise or activity. • If the child needs to hum to concentrate, teach the child to hum more quietly. • Allow the child to use and play with "vibration" by using such items as an electric toothbrush or a kazoo.
Is bothered by the noises of household appliances.	• Sometimes the pitch and frequency of household appliances can be very distracting and annoying to children who experience auditory issues.	• Expose the child to the "irritating" noise in small steps, gradually increasing the duration as tolerance improves. • Warn the child that the appliance is going to be turned on so she won't be taken by surprise. • Have the child participate in using the appliance, if appropriate. • Lessen the unpleasant effect of the noise by combining it with pleasant sound (music on the radio). • Pair the noise with a preferred activity.
Notices every little sound or visual change in the environment.	• These distractions can be overwhelming, making it difficult for the child to remain focused.	• Keep visual/auditory distractions to a minimum. • Set up a quiet place with a bean bag chair for the child. • Consider alternate seating away from distractions. • Prepare the child in advance for distractions such as announcements or visitors, using a visual support that reflects the anticipated change. • Consider using a visual barrier or "cubicle" for desk work. • Provide headphones or earplugs for the child to wear during testing or seatwork after verbal directives are given.

Table 4.2 (continued)

Incident	Interpretation	Intervention
NOISE/SOUND (continued)		
Talks self through a task.	• May need the added input to help keep himself focused and stay on task to completion. • Sound of own voice may block out other auditory input. • May have poor self-concept about abilities based on motor planning difficulties.	• Allow the child to do this if it does not interfere with others. • Utilize a hand fidget to help decrease anxiety or enhance self-regulation. • Provide a weighted lap pad for deep pressure input. • Develop visual supports for use in a situation where child is unable to talk himself through tasks without disturbing others. This might also give him the extra support to refocus and continue if he becomes distracted. • Teach the child to self-talk using a lower volume or standing away from others.
ORGANIZATION		
Has poor organizational skills; constantly loses school materials; papers fall out of notebook.	• Has difficulty focusing on relevant stimuli. • Has difficulty discriminating the items he may need from other things in his desk.	• Provide visual structure through color coding or assignment books. • Use tape inside the desk as a boundary marker for books. • Organize materials under the desk or on a bookshelf so they are always visible. • Use a sturdy box lid to contain student materials. Slide the box into the desk where it serves as a laptop desk. • Provide a notebook to carry papers to and from home with clearly marked "Homework" sections for each subject.
Talks self through a task.	• May need the added input to help keep himself focused and stay on task to completion. • Sound of own voice may block out other auditory input. • May have poor self-concept about abilities based on motor planning difficulties.	• Allow the child to do this if it does not interfere with others. • Utilize a hand fidget to help decrease anxiety. • Provide a weighted lap pad for deep pressure input. • Develop visual supports for use in a situation where child is unable to talk himself through tasks without disturbing others. This might also give him the extra support to refocus and continue if he becomes distracted. • Teach the child to self-talk using a lower volume.

Table 4.2 (continued)

Incident	Interpretation	Intervention
PLAY		
Engages in rough play during recess, gym class, and organized sport activities.	• Has unclear understanding of own strength. • Seeks proprioceptive input. • May not be able to judge where her body is in relation to other children.	• Prior to contact sports, have the child participate in gross-motor activities (i.e., jumping, wheelbarrow races, crab crawls, tug-of-war) that increase body awareness. • Have the child wear a compression-type garment (Spandex™ or Lycra™) under regular clothes. • Make recess a series of planned activities that look like an obstacle course, including hanging by hands or feet, pushing, pulling, or jumping.
Is hesitant to access playground equipment or participate in games and play where feet lose contact with the ground.	• May be afraid of falling and needs the reassurance of being connected to the ground.	• Allow the child to direct the movement initially. • Grade the activity to a level with less challenge or threat to the child. • Provide supervised practice opportunities in advance of participation in the activity with others. • Incorporate additional proprioceptive stimulation with weight or tactile input by briskly rubbing prior to activity.
ROUTINES		
Experiences difficulty when changes occur.	• A routine provides predictability and helps stay organized and focused. • Needs predictability, especially if his body does not "feel in control." • Feels the need to structure schedules and activities to avoid unpleasant sensory experiences. • Does not know what to do when change occurs.	• Offer the child a signal before a change occurs. • Prepare the child for changes using visual supports. • Give the child a script to use when an unexpected event occurs. • Gradually incorporate "unplanned" activities into the schedule, starting with preferred activities. • Incorporate a "change" symbol into the child's schedule.
Has rigid rituals at home and school.	• Prefers to have predictability in his environment. • Feels the need to structure schedule and activities to avoid unpleasant sensory experiences. • Motor planning challenges motivate the child to engage only in activities he feels competent about.	• Honor the ritual whenever possible if it doesn't interfere with daily living activities. • Use visual supports/schedules to help the child to stay organized. • Make changes in the "usual" scheduling and offer strategies that the child can use to help him cope with these changes. • Elaborate on the child's ritual by altering one sensory aspect at a time as a way to introduce flexibility. An example might be using a strong-scented or granular soap during a hand-washing routine. • Warn the child ahead of time that the ritual may be different. • Offer a quiet place for the child to help him calm down or reorganize. • Allow the child access to a swing or rocking chair.

Table 4.2 (continued)

Incident	Interpretation	Intervention
SITTING		
Crawls under desk.	• Needs to be away from distractions from others talking, lights buzzing, etc. • Needs her personal space defined.	• Provide a quiet area in the room for the child. The area could contain beanbags, large pillows, or a rocking chair. • Reinforce with positive feedback when the child lets you know he needs some "quiet time." • Provide a large barrel or small playhouse for sitting. • Wrap the child in a quilt. • Allow the child to sit in an upholstered chair with arm rests. • Seat the child away from distractors. • Seat the child near the teacher.
Has difficulty keeping hands and feet to self when sitting in groups.	• Craves tactile input. • Doesn't understand about personal boundaries. • May learn by handling or manipulating objects.	• Provide visual or physical boundaries for sitting such as tape boundaries, carpet squares, placemats, inflatable disc, or camping pillow. • Provide a "fidget item" such as a Koosh Ball™ or Tangle™. Often fidget items can be academically related, such as holding a play cow when studying farm animals or grasping a squeeze/stress ball that looks like a planet when studying the solar system. • If the reaction occurs during a floor-based activity, have child lie on her stomach, propping her head on her elbows. • Have a child hold or squeeze a large pillow held in lap.
Sits with legs on top of chair back.	• Desk and chair may not fit student size. • May need additional proprioceptive input. May be self-regulating.	• If the child is not in danger of hurting himself, allow the behavior. • Ensure that desk and chair size are appropriate for child. • Provide inflatable disc, camping pillow, therapy ball or t-stool. • Allow the child to complete assignments while lying on the floor or standing by the desk. • Have the child sit on her legs. • Give frequent movement breaks.

Table 4.2 *(continued)*

Incident	Interpretation	Intervention
SLEEPING		
Is a very restless sleeper.	• May be uncomfortable with the sheets on her bed as the light touch may be more irritating than calming. • May become distracted by light or noise while trying to sleep. • May not require "standard" amount of sleep due to medications or natural constitution. • May have difficulty with self-regulation.	• Have the child sleep in a sleeping bag and/or under a comforter. • Warm bedclothes in dryer. • Try using flannel sheets because cotton sheets often form little "pills" that may be irritating. • Before bedtime, rub the child with lotion or powder. This may be calming to her system, helping her to settle down to sleep. • What the child wears to bed might also impact her ability to sleep comfortably. Some children prefer heavy, tight-fitting pajamas, while others are more comfortable in a light-weight t-shirt. • Consider that children benefit from enclosing their bed in a tent-like manner to filter out light and noises. • Try to establish a predictable routine for bedtime. • Be aware that roughhouse play can be helpful to prepare them for sleep. For others it may be overstimulating. • Consider giving the child a warm bath or shower prior to bedtime. • Try white noise as a way to calm the child. A fan or relaxing music may aid in sleep. • Provide water bottle with straw to drink at night if needed.
Prefers sleeping on the floor instead of bed.	• May prefer to remain close to the ground. • May not be comfortable in his bed because of the mattress or sheets.	• Allow the child to sleep on the floor in a sleeping bag. • Try placing the child's mattress on the floor. • Use flannel sheets, a sleeping bag, or heavy comforter. • Provide the child with a body pillow or stuffed animal.
TOUCHING		
Avoids messy materials such as paints, glue, shaving cream.	• Activities involving certain kinds of materials may be uncomfortable for the child.	• Encourage tolerance (without forcing) of these kinds of materials through controlled, gradual exposure to various items and textures. • Prepare the child for a given activity by providing a visual cue. • Plan activities that are uncomfortable followed by activities that the child likes. As the activity becomes more tolerable, gradually increase the length of time child is engaged in it.

Table 4.2 (continued)

Incident	Interpretation	Intervention
TOUCHING (continued)		
Drags hands along walls when walking.	• Seeks tactile input. • Needs proprioceptive input to help him feel comfortable. • May like the feel of the wall.	• Allow the child to do it. • Have the child carry something that has a texture and surface similar to the wall. • If the child is young, have her hold the hand of a peer or adult. • Have the child hold on to a rope or classroom object. • Have the child carry a container holding the materials to be used in the next class or activity. • Provide proprioceptive or vestibular input by having the child hop, skip, do jumping jacks, or bend down and touch toes half way down the hall. • Instruct the child to carry her books against her body with hands touching opposite elbows.
Picks at scabs, lips and nose.	• May be anxious. • Reaction may calm and aid concentration. • Input may help increase alertness if the child is bored with surroundings. • Increased attention to a skin breakdown in various stages of healing may come from an itching or irritating tactile sensation.	• Provide fidget items such as Koosh Ball™, therapy putty, pliable art eraser, bookmark with a tassel, small toys or manipulatives. • Place a strip of Velcro™ (one or both sides) inside book binder or underneath the desk that the child can play with or pick at. • Use topical ointments or lubricants that may help to alleviate or alter the irritating sensory input.
Touches everything.	• May learn through touching. • May desire more tactile input.	• When possible, allow the child to explore. • Before the child enters the environment in which there are many items that are not to be touched, provide deep pressure by rubbing shoulders, back, or palms. • Accompany a touch by a verbal statement of the rules for touching. • Allow the child to hold an object that can provide deep pressure.

Table 4.2 (continued)

Incident	Interpretation	Intervention
WRITING/COLORING		
Has messy handwriting; unable to stay within the lines.	• Does not receive the appropriate sensations to plan how to move and design a sequence of what comes next. • Feel of the pencil may interfere with an effective pencil grasp. • Creative writing or generating own sentences is more challenging than copying.	• Have the child engage in gross-motor activities before he is asked to perform fine-motor activities such as 5 chair push-ups or donkey kicks before writing. • Encourage the child to participate in activities that develop hand strength (i.e., wheelbarrow walking, crawling). • Hide items in therapy putty and ask the child to find them. This can be made more challenging by asking the child to do the activity using only one hand to pull the putty apart to retrieve the small items inside. • Emphasize movement with handwriting instruction, such as practicing large letters in the air or on the chalkboard. • Have the child write on "bumpy" paper with raised lines.
Holds pencils and crayons by fingertips only and only uses fingertips when feeling toys.	• Touching items with the palm of the hand may be uncomfortable. • May not have the appropriate amount of strength in her hands.	• Provide deep pressure input (using thumb to rub) to palm of child's hand prior to activity. • Encourage activities that require the hands to touch and hold materials and objects such as constructing toys and art projects. • Incorporate various textures during play such as beans or rice. • Use activities that progress from only using fingertips to involving the whole hand. Introduce finger paints, shaving cream and lotion first. Then move to activities requiring hands, such as holding a ball or playing with Playdoh™.

Summary

Children and youth with HF-ASD have complex needs. Strategies that are effective one day may not work the next. In addition, some strategies may not be appropriate at all for a given child or student. Due to the complexities of these issues, consider tolerating sensory behaviors that are not keeping the child from participating in daily activities or disrupting others, thereby respecting the child's preferences and individual sensory systems. Occupational therapists and others trained in sensory integration techniques can provide valuable assistance in selecting and using strategies. Be creative and trust your instincts. Be a detective, but don't spend so much time analyzing behaviors that you miss opportunities to enjoy the child's individuality. By using the information and suggestions presented in this book, you can help the child with HF-ASD "make sense" of the world.

CHAPTER 5

MEETING CHILDREN'S SENSORY NEEDS ACROSS THE DAY AND ACROSS ENVIRONMENTS

Sensory issues occur throughout the day and throughout the multiple environments in which we participate. Thus, it is essential that all interventions and supports are embedded within the routines and activities that are part of the learner's day to facilitate the best possible access to learning opportunities and to promote generalization (Barton, Lawrence, & Deurloo, 2012; Boulware, Schwartz, Sandall, & McBride, 2006; Kurth & Mastergeorge, 2010; Schertz, Baker, Hurwitz, & Benner, 2011; Witt, VanDerHeyden, & Gilbertson, 2004; Woods & Brown, 2011).

Several systems have been developed to help ensure that interventions are entrenched into the daily schedule – whether at home, school, work, or community. These include the Comprehensive Autism Planning System (CAPS) (Henry & Myles, 2013), the Ziggurat Model (Aspy & Grossman, 2011), the Out and About Model (Hudson & Coffin, 2007), and the Destination Friendship Model (Benton, Hollis, Mahler, & Womer, 2011).

Each of these practical models will be discussed below.

The Comprehensive Autism Planning System (CAPS)

Developed by Henry and Myles (2013), the CAPS provides an overview of the student's daily schedule by time and activity as well as the supports the student needs across the day. CAPS can be used in:

- Home
- School
- Community
- Workplace

Because it is suitable across the lifespan and across environments and lists (a) the skills to be taught, (b) data collection parameters, as well as (c) when supports are needed, the CAPS is often referred to as the implementation arm of the IEP or the "practical IEP."

As illustrated in Figure 5.1, part of the CAPS includes a detailed analysis of the learner's day; a listing of supports, skills to teach, data collection, and generalization information for each daily activity; and photographs of each support.

CAPS answers the following important questions:

1. What supports should be embedded into the individual's daily activities to support optimal learning and performance?

2. What information can I pass on to the adults who will support the individual in the future to ensure that the person's interventions and strategies that promoted success are clearly understood?

The Comprehensive Autism Planning System (CAPS)

Child/Student:

Time	Activity	Targeted Skills to Teach	Structure/ Modifications	Reinforcement	Sensory Strategies	Communication Social Skills	Data Collection	Generalization Plan
8:00	Reading	Common Core	Vocabulary cards Bookmark	Verbal Book on apes (interest)	None			
8:50	Math	Common Core	1/2 problems Timer Test in resource room	Verbal Computer when done	Earbuds for independent work Breaks			

- Headphones
- Brief break
- Baseball caps
- iPod with music
- Self-regulation scale
- Incredible 5-Point Scale
- And so forth

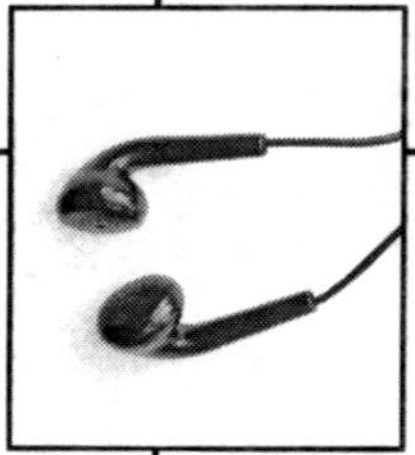

Figure 5.1. The Comprehensive Autism Planning System (CAPS).

The Ziggurat Model

The Ziggurat Model is a comprehensive planning model for individuals with ASD across the spectrum and across the lifespan based on the premise that in order for a program to be successful for an individual with ASD, his unique needs and strengths must be identified and then directly linked to interventions (Aspy & Grossman, 2011). Therefore, the Ziggurat Model utilizes students' strengths to address true needs or underlying deficits that result in social, emotional, and behavioral concerns. In doing so, the Ziggurat approach centers on a hierarchical system consisting of five levels: Sensory Differences and Biological Needs, Reinforcement, Structure and Visual/Tactile Supports, Task Demands, and Skills to Teach that must be addressed for an intervention plan to be comprehensive (see Figure 5.2).

The first and foundational level, Sensory Differences and Biological Needs, addresses basic internal factors that impact functioning. The second level addresses motivational needs prerequisite to skill development. The third level draws on individuals' strength of visual processing and addresses their fundamental need for order and routine. The final two levels of the Ziggurat emphasize the importance of expectations and skill development relative to the characteristics of individuals with ASD.

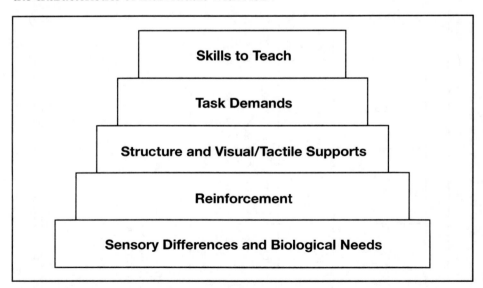

Figure 5.2. The five levels of the Ziggurat Model.

From Aspy, R., & Grossman, B. G. (2011). *Designing comprehensive interventions for high-functioning individuals with autism spectrum disorders: The Ziggurat Model – Release 2.0.* Shawnee Mission, KS: AAPC Publishing. Used with permission.

Traditional views of program planning often focus on interventions that address only surface or observable behavior without consideration of underlying ASD characteristics. These are potentially less effective and, therefore, less likely to result in sustained behavior change. The Ziggurat Model is different. By targeting an individual's specific needs, defined by ASD characteristics, it leads to interventions that are proactive and effective. The model can be used in two ways: (a) as a global planning tool for school, home, workplace, and/or community; or (b) as a functional behavior assessment. A complete discussion of the Ziggurat Model is beyond the scope of this book, but Figure 5.3 shows the process. In addition, the CAPS model can be integrated into the Ziggurat Model.

Ziggurat Worksheet		CAPS
Skills to Teach	→	Targeted Skills to Teach
Structure and Visual/Tactile Supports Task Demands Skills to Teach	→	Structure/Modifications
Reinforcement Structure and Visual/Tactile Supports	→	Reinforcement
Sensory and Biological Task Demands Skills to Teach	→	Sensory Strategies
Sensory and Biological Structure and Visual/Tactile Supports Task Demands Skills to Teach	→	Communication/Social Skills

Figure 5.3. The Ziggurat Model process.

From Aspy, R., & Grossman, B. G. (2011). *Designing comprehensive interventions for high-functioning individuals with autism spectrum disorders: The Ziggurat Model – Release 2.0.* Shawnee Mission, KS: AAPC Publishing. Used with permission.

The Out and About Model

The Out and About Blueprint (Hudson & Coffin, 2007) was developed to help individuals with ASD have successful community outings. Designed to be completed by a caregiver and/or professional who accompanies a child on a community outing, it is reviewed with the learner prior to the event. The form's Rewind box is a place for making notes about what went well and what could be changed or adapted for another similar outing in the future, because even with the best planning, not all outings are successful each time.

Figure 5.4 provides an Out and About Blueprint for LaBrahn, who was going on a field trip to a pizza restaurant with his classmates.

SUPPORT	STRATEGY	DESIRED OUTCOME
Waiting plan	Use 5,4,3,2,1 cards; chat with the group	Visual countdown will help cope with waiting
Communication	Use AAC device preprogrammed for outing	Ordering independently
Social	Create social narrative with AAC icons and words – one concept per page	Advance information about environment and expectations of trip
Visual	Prepare single-step cards of event to use while at restaurant	Controlling anxiety and providing predictability
Hidden curriculum	Emphasize reminder phrase: "We do not touch other people's hats"	Keeping hands to himself
Sensory	Bring lap weight to hold while sitting at table; tennis balls for rocking; break card	Self-regulation
Motivation	Remind "First pizza . . . Then video games"	Attending to task
Behavior	—	—
Transition	Add visual icon on daily schedule; use countdown until time to leave	Going and returning with ease
For sibling or other students	—	—

Additional activities for school:
Practice with AAC device; role-play sequence of events

Additional activities for home:
Use AAC device to request and comment on items during dinner

REWIND
Difficult time transitioning from video games when it was time to leave

Suggestion for next time: emphasize transition to leave in social narrative, highlighting transition cue

Figure 5.4. The Out and About Model Blueprint.

From Hudson, J., & Coffin, A. B. (2007). *Out and About: Preparing Children With Autism Spectrum Disorders to Participate in Their Communities*. Shawnee Mission, KS: AAPC Publishing. Reprinted with permission.

The Destination Friendship Model

The Destination Friendship Model (Benton et al., 2011) provides a step-by-step guide to providing friendship groups. The model is very different from traditional social skill group models by using motivating, fun activities that kids 'typically' do and subtly infuses strategies and supports directly within these activities. No lessons or contrived activities. Just everyday fun like playing video games, cooking, singing karaoke, eating pizza, swimming, and participating in ping pong tournaments. It is all the work behind the scenes that makes Destination Friendship successful. In order to provide these opportunities for children with HF-ASD to get together, feel celebrated, and have typical, fun childhood experiences, it is important to proactively embed supports, however concealed they may be, to ensure successful participation.

The Friendship Skills Checklist, which is an important part of The Destination Friendship Model, is used to glean information regarding the underlying strengths and needs of each participant. The checklist, which looks at 13 Core Skill Areas, takes into account the typical skill difficulties experienced by individuals with HF-ASD. Once a caregiver completes the checklist, the information is used by the leaders to decide how to utilize areas of strength and proactively select strategies that "secretly" target and/or support the areas of need. These strategies are then embedded continuously throughout the entire group experience

The Destination Friendship Model stresses the importance of effective self-regulation skills and the impact that self-regulation or lack thereof can have on the ability to make and keep friends. One of the three areas of Self-Regulation addressed by the Destination Friendship Model is Sensory Regulation (see Figure 5.5). Once the caregiver completes the Friendship Skill Checklist and an overview of the child's Sensory Regulation needs is gleaned, the leaders plan proactively how to support these areas of challenge. The leaders can choose from a variety of Sensory Regulation strategies provided or create their own strategies. Either way the model promotes the importance of embedding these strategies directly within the fun activities to promote success.

Friendship Skills Checklist

Directions: Please think about the individual in a variety of settings (home, school, community) when completing this questionnaire. When reading each question, rate your response according to the following scale: M = Mostly (this skill is observed greater than 75% of the time across environments), O = Often (this skill is observed 25% to 75% of the time across environments), R = Rarely (this skill is observed less than 25% of the time across environments).

Information on Friends

Does the individual have friends? (check) ☐ Yes ☐ No

How many friends does your individual have? (check) ☐ 0-2 ☐ 2-4 ☐ 5 +

Are they friends from (check): ☐ School ☐ Community ☐ Other:

Does the individual get together with these friends? (check) ☐ Yes ☐ No

How often does the individual get together with friends? (check) ☐ Daily ☐ Weekly ☐ Monthly

Does the individual express a desire to have friends? (check) ☐ Yes ☐ No

Is the individual content with having or not having friends? (check) ☐ Yes ☐ No

List any situations or activities in which the individual socially excels (i.e., sporting activity, job, etc.).

List any frustrations regarding friendships identified by the individual:

Questions	M	O	R
SELF-REGULATION			
Sensory Regulation			
Can the individual effectively tolerate sensory input? Circle any that are difficult: Touch, Sound, Crowds, Visual.			
Can the individual appropriately express sensory discomfort (tell someone he is too close, ask for quiet, etc.)?			
Does the individual respect personal space/boundaries?			

Key: **M** = Mostly; **O** = Occasionally; **R** = Rarely.

Figure 5.5. Friendship Skills Checklist.

From Benton, M., Hollis, C., Mahler, K., & Womer, A. (2011). *Destination Friendship*. Shawnee Mission, KS: AAPC Publishing. Reprinted with permission.

Summary

Sensory-based interventions can be extremely helpful when included as a part of daily routines. The CAPS, Ziggurat Model, the Out and About template, and the Destination Friendship Model all help ensure that this happens.

We now understand a lot more about individuals with HF-ASD, but we have a long way to go. Sensory issues are well established as a common cause of the challenges experienced by persons with HF-ASD. We hope this book serves as a good summary of these sensory issues and allows the reader to implement supports that maximize comfort and success.

REFERENCES

Adamson, A., O'Hare, A., & Graham, C. (2006). Impairments in sensory modulation in children with autistic spectrum disorder. *British Journal of Occupational Therapy, 69,* 357-364.

American Psychiatric Association. (2013). *Diagnostic and statistical manual of mental disorders* (5th ed.). Arlington, VA: Author.

Ashwin, E., Ashwin, C., Rhydderch, D., Howells, J., & Baron-Cohen, S. (2009). Eagle-eyed visual acuity: An experimental investigation of enhanced perception in autism. *Biological Psychiatry, 65*(1), 17-21.

Asperger, H. (1994). Autistic psychopathy in childhood (U. Frith, Trans.). In U. Frith (Ed.), *Autism and Asperger syndrome* (pp. 37-92). New York, NY: Cambridge University Press. (Original work published 1944).

Aspy, R., & Grossman, B. G. (2011). *Designing comprehensive interventions for high-functioning individuals with autism spectrum disorders: The Ziggurat Model – Release 2.0.* Shawnee Mission, KS: AAPC Publishing.

Ayres, A. J. (1972). *Sensory integration and learning disorders.* Los Angeles, CA: Western Psychological Services.

Ayres, A. J. (1979). *Sensory integration and the child.* Los Angeles, CA: Western Psychological Services.

Ayres, A. J. (1989). *The sensory integration and praxis tests.* Los Angeles, CA: Western Psychological Services.

Baker, A.E.Z., Lane, A., Angley, M. T., & Young, R. L. (2008). The relationship between sensory processing patterns and behavioral responsiveness in autistic disorder: A pilot study. *Journal of Autism and Developmental Disorders, 38,* 867-875.

Baranek, G., David, F. J., Poe, M. D., Stone, W. L., & Watson, L. R. (2006). Sensory experiences questionnaire: Discriminating features in young children with autism, developmental delays, and typical development. *Journal of Child Psychology and Psychiatry & Allied Disciplines, 47*(6), 591-601.

Barton, E. E., Lawrence, K., & Deurloo, F. (2012). Individualizing interventions for young children with autism in preschool. *Journal of Autism and Developmental Disorders, 42,* 1205-1217.

Bennetto, L., Kuschner, E. S., & Hyman, S. L. (2007). Olfaction and taste processing in autism. *Biological Psychiatry, 62*(9), 1015-1021.

Benton, M., Hollis, C., Mahler, K., & Womer, A. (2011). *Destination friendship: Developing social skills for individuals with autism spectrum disorder or other social challenges.* Shawnee Mission, KS: AAPC Publishing.

Ben-Sasson, A., Hen, L., Fluss, R., Cermak, S. A., Engel-Yeger, B., & Gal, E. (2009). A metaanalysis of sensory modulation symptoms with autism spectrum disorders. *Journal of Autism and Developmental Disorders, 39*, 1-11.

Blakemore, S. J., Tavassoli, T., Calò, S., Thomas, R. M., Catmur, C., Frith, U., & Haggard, P. (2006). *Tactile sensitivity in Asperger syndrome. Brain and Cognition, 61*(1), 5-13.

Blanche, E., & Schaaf, R. (2001). Proprioception: A cornerstone of sensory integrative intervention. In S. Roley, E. Blanche, & R. Schaaf (Eds.), *Understanding the nature of sensory integration with diverse populations* (pp. 109-131). San Antonio, TX: Psychological Corporation.

Boulware, G., Schwartz, I. S., Sandall, S. R., & McBride, B. J. (2006). Project DATA for toddlers: An inclusive approach to very young children with autism spectrum disorder. *Topics in Early Childhood Special Education, 26*(2), 94-105.

Brack, J. C. (2004). *Learn to move, move to learn: Sensorimotor early childhood activity themes.* Shawnee Mission, KS: AAPC Publishing.

Brack, J. C. (2005). *Learn to move, move to learn, dinosaurs.* Shawnee Mission, KS: AAPC Publishing.

Brack, J. C. (2006). *Sensory processing disorder: Simulations and solutions for parents, teachers, and therapists [DVD and kit].* Shawnee Mission, KS: AAPC Publishing.

Brack, J. C. (2009). *Learn to move, moving up! Sensorimotor elementary-school activity themes.* Shawnee Mission, KS: AAPC Publishing.

Brown, C., & Dunn, W. (2002). *Adolescent/Adult Sensory Profile manual.* San Antonio, TX: Psychological Corporation.

Buie, T., Campbell, D. B., Fuchs, G. J., III, Furuta, J., Levy, J., VandeWater, A. H., Winter, H., et al. (2010). Evaluation, diagnoses, and treatment of gastrointestinal disorders in individuals with ASDs: A consensus report. *Pediatrics, 125* (Suppl.), S1-S29.

Buron, K. D. (2007). *A "5" could make me lose control: An activity-based method for evaluating and supporting highly anxious students.* Shawnee Mission, KS: AAPC Publishing.

Buron, K. D., & Curtis, M. B. (2012). *The incredible 5-point scale: The significantly improved and expanded second edition; Assisting students in understanding social interactions and controlling their emotional responses.* Shawnee Mission, KS: AAPC Publishing.

Buron, K. D. (2013). *When my worries get too big! A relaxation book for children who live with anxiety – Revised and expanded edition.* Shawnee Mission, KS: AAPC Publishing.

Centers for Medicare and Medicaid Services. (2010). *Autism spectrum disorders: Final report on environmental scan.* Washington, DC: Author.

Cermak, S. A., Curtin, C., & Bandini, L. G. (2010). Food selectivity and sensory sensitivity in children with autism spectrum disorders. *Journal of the American Dietetic Association, 110*(2), 238-246. doi:10.1016/j.jada.2009.10.032

Chang, M C., Parham, L. D., Blanche, E. L., Schell, A., Chou, C. P., Dawson, M., & Clark, F. (2012). Autonomic and behavioral responses of children with autism to auditory stimuli. *The American Journal of Occupational Therapy, 66*(5), 567-576.

Craig, A. D. (2002). How do you feel? Interoception: The sense of the physiological condition of the body. *Nature Reviews Neuroscience, 3,* 655-666.

Craig, A. D. (2003). Interoception: The sense of the physiological condition of the body. *Current Opinion in Neurobiology, 13*(4), 500-505.

Culp, S. (2011). *A buffet of sensory interventions: Solutions for middle and high school students.* Shawnee Mission, KS: AAPC Publishing.

Devlin, S., Leader, G., & Healy, O. (2009). Comparison of behavioral intervention and sensory integration therapy in the treatment of self-injurious behavior. *Research in Autism Spectrum Disorders, 3,* 223-231.

Dunn, W. (1997). The impact of sensory processing abilities on the daily lives of young children and their families: A conceptual model. *Infants and Young Children, 9*(4), 23-25.

Dunn, W. (1999). *The Sensory Profile.* San Antonio, TX: Therapy Skill Builders.

Dunn, W. (2002). *Infant Toddler Sensory Profile manual.* San Antonio, TX: Psychological Corporation.

Dunn, W. (2006). *Sensory Profile-School Companion manual.* San Antonio, TX: Psychological Corporation.

Dunn, W., Myles, B. S., & Orr, S. (2002). Sensory processing issues associated with Asperger syndrome: A preliminary investigation. *American Journal of Occupational Therapy, 56*(1), 97-102.

Endow, J. (2009). *Outsmarting explosive behavior: A visual system of support and intervention for individuals with autism spectrum disorders.* Shawnee Mission, KS: AAPC Publishing.

Falkmer, M., Stuart, G. W., Danielsson, H., Bram, S., Lönebrink, M., & Falkmer, T. (2011). Visual acuity in adults with Asperger's syndrome: No evidence for "eagle-eyed" vision. *Biological Psychiatry, 70*(9), 812-816.

Fazlioğlu, Y., & Baran, G. (2008). A sensory integration therapy program on sensory problems for children with autism. *Perceptual Motor Skills, 106*(2), 415-422.

Fuentes, C. T., Mostofsky, S. H., & Bastian, A. J. (2011). No proprioceptive deficits in autism despite movement related sensory and execution impairments. *Journal of Autism and Developmental Disorders, 41,* 1352-1361. doi.org/10.1007/s10803-010-1161-1

Goldsmith, H. H., Van Hulle, C. A., Arneson, C. L., Schreiber, J. E., & Gernsbacher, M. A. (2006). A population-based twin study of parentally reported tactile and auditory defensiveness in young children. *Journal of Abnormal Child Psychology, 34*(3), 393-407.

Grandin, T. (1996). *Thinking in pictures.* Vancouver, WA: Vintage Books.

Groen, W. B., Zwiers, M. P., van der Gaag, R. J., & Buitelaar, J. K. (2008). The phenotype and neural correlates of language in autism: An integrative review. *Neuroscience & Biobehavioral Reviews, 32,* 1416-1425.

Güclü, B., Tanidir, C., Mukaddes. N. M., & Unal, F. (2007). Tactile sensitivity of normal and autistic children. *Somantosensory and Motor Research, 24*(1-2), 21-33, 13, 5.

Henry, D. (1998). *Tool chest for teachers, parents, and students: A handbook to facilitate self-regulation.* Youngtown, AZ: Henry Occupational Therapy Services.

Henry, S. A., & Myles, B. S. (2013). *The comprehensive autism planning system (CAPS) for individuals with autism spectrum disorders and related disabilities: Integrating evidence-based practices throughout the student's day* (2nd ed.). Shawnee Mission, KS: AAPC Publishing.

Hilton, C. L., Harper, J. D., Kueker, R. H., Lang, A. R., Abbachhi, A. M., Todorov, A., & LaVesser, P. D. (2010). Sensory responsiveness as a predictor of social severity in children with high functioning autism spectrum disorders. *Journal of Autism and Developmental Disorders, 40,* 937-945.

Hrdlicka, M., Vodicka, J., Havlovicova, M., Urbanek, T., Blatny, M., & Dudova, I. (2011). Brief report: Significant differences in perceived odor pleasantness found in children with ASD. *Journal of Autism and Developmental Disorders, 41,* 524-527.

Hudson, J., & Coffin, A. B. (2007). *Out and about: Preparing children with autism spectrum disorders to participate in their communities.* Shawnee Mission, KS: AAPC Publishing.

Källstrand, J., Olsson, O., Nehlstedt, S. F., Sköld, M. L., & Nielzén, S. (2010). Abnormal auditory forward masking pattern in the brainstem response of individuals with Asperger syndrome. *Neuropsychiatry Diseases and Treatment, 6,* 289-296.

Kanner, L. (1943). Autistic disturbances of affective contact. *The Nervous Child, 2,* 217-250.

Kern, J. K., Garver, C. R., Carmody, T., Andres, A. A., Mehta, J. A., & Trivedi, M. H. (2008). Examining sensory modulation in individuals with autism as compared to community controls. *Research in Autism Spectrum Disorders, 2,* 85-94.

Kern, J. K., Garver, C. R., Grannemann, B. D., Trivedi, M. H., Carmody, T., Andrews, A. A., et al. (2007). Response to vestibular sensory events in autism. *Research in Autism Spectrum Disorders, 1,* 67-74.

Kerstein, L. (2008). *My sensory book: Working together to explore sensory issues and the big feelings they can cause: A workbook for parents, professionals, and children.* Shawnee Mission, KS: AAPC Publishing.

Kienz, K., & Miller, H. (1999, March). Classroom evaluation of the child with autism. School System. *Special Interest Section Quarterly, 6*(1), 4.

Kurth, J., & Mastergeorge, A. M. (2010). Individual education plan goals and services for adolescents with autism: Impact of age and educational setting. *The Journal of Special Education, 44*(3), 146-160.

Kwakye, L. D., Foss-Feig, J. H., Cascio, C. J., Stone, W. L., & Wallace, M. T. (2011). Altered auditory and multisensory temporal processing in autism spectrum disorders. *Frontiers in Integrative Neuroscience, 4,* 129. doi:10.3389/fnint.2010.00129

Kwon, S., Kim, J., Choe, B. H., Ko, C., & Park, S. (2007). Electrophysiologic assessment of central auditory processing by auditory brainstem responses in children with autism spectrum disorders. *Journal of Korean Medical Science, 22,* 656-659.

Lane, A. E., Young, R. L., Baker, A. E., & Angley, M. T. (2010). Sensory processing subtypes in autism: Association with adaptive behavior. *Journal of Autism and Developmental Disorders, 40*(1), 112-122. doi:10.1007/s10803-009-0840-2.

Larson, E. M. (2008). *The Chameleon Kid: Controlling Meltdown before he controls you.* Shawnee Mission, KS: AAPC Publishing.

Leekam, S. R., Nieto, C., Libby, S. J., Wing, L., & Gould, J. (2007). Describing the sensory abnormalities of children and adults with autism. *Journal of Autism and Developmental Disorders, 37*, 894-910.

Lowrence, L. (1994). *Techniques and suggestions for evaluating persons with autism.* Paper presented at the meeting of the Autism Society of America Convention Kansas City, MO.

Mahler, K. (2009). *Hygiene and related behaviors for children and adolescents with autism spectrum and related disorders: A fun curriculum with a focus on social understanding.* Shawnee Mission, KS: AAPC Publishing.

Manasco, H. (2006). *The way to A: Empowering children with autism spectrum and other neurological disorders to monitor and replace aggression and tantrum behavior.* Shawnee Mission, KS: AAPC Publishing.

Marco, E. J., Hinkley, L.B.N., Hill, S. S., & Nagarajan, S. S. (2011). Sensory processing in autism: A review of neurophysiologic findings. *Pediatric Research, 69*(5), 48R-54R.

Mayes, L. (2000). A developmental perspective on the regulation of arousal states. *Seminars in Perinatology, 24*(4), 267-279. doi:10.1053/sper.2000.9121

McIntosh, D. N., Miller, L. J., Shyu, V., & Dunn, W. (1999). Overview of the Short Sensory Profile (SSP). In W. Dunn (Ed.), *The Sensory Profile: Examiner's manual* (pp. 59-73). San Antonio, TX: Psychological Corporation.

Miller, L. J. (2006). *Sensational kids: Help and hope for children with sensory processing disorder.* New York, NY: Putnam.

Miller, L. J., Anzalone, M. E., Lane, S. J., Cermak, S. A., & Osten, E. T. (2007). Concept evolution in sensory integration. A proposed nosology for diagnosis. *American Journal of Occupational Therapy, 61*, 135-140.

Miller-Kuhaneck, H., Ecker, C., Parham, L. D., Henry, D. A., & Glennon, T. J. (2010). *Sensory Processing Measure Preschool (SPM-P): Manual.* Los Angeles, CA: Western Psychological Services.

Miller-Kuhaneck, H., Henry, D. & Glennon, T. (2007). *The Sensory Processing Measure – Main Classroom and School Environments.* Los Angeles, CA: Western Psychological Services.

Molloy, C. A., Dietrich, K. N., & Bhattacharya, A. (2003). Postural stability in children with autism spectrum disorder. *Journal of Autism and Developmental Disorders, 33*, 643-652.

Mostofsky, S. H., & Ewen, J. B. (2011). Altered connectivity and action model formation in autism is autism. *The Neuroscientist, 17*, 437-448.

Moyer, S., & NHS. (2009). *The ECLIPSE model: Teaching self-regulation, executive function, attribution, and sensory awareness to students with Asperger syndrome, high-functioning autism, and related disorders.* Shawnee Mission, KS: AAPC Publishing.

Myles, B. S., Hagiwara, T., Dunn, W., Rinner, L., Reese, M., Huggins, A., & Becker, S. (2004). Sensory issues in children with Asperger Syndrome and autism. *Education and Training in Developmental Disabilities, 3*(4), 283-290.

Myles, B. S., Lee, H. J., Smith, S. M., Tien, K., Chou, Y., Swanson, T. C., & Hudson, J. (2007). A large-scale study of the characteristics of Asperger Syndrome. *Education and Training in Developmental Disabilities, 42*(4), 448-459.

Myles, B. S., & Southwick, J. (2005). *Asperger syndrome and difficult moments: Practical solutions for tantrums, rage, and meltdowns* (2nd ed.). Shawnee Mission, KS: AAPC Publishing.

National Autism Center (NAC). (2009). *National standards report: Addressing the need for evidence-based practice guidelines for autism spectrum disorders.* Randolph, MA: Author.

National Professional Development Center on Autism Spectrum Disorders (NPDC on ASD). (2009). *Evidence-based practice briefs.* Retrieved from http://autismpdc.fpg.unc.edu/content/briefs.

Parham, L. D., & Ecker, C. (2007). *Sensory processing measure-home form.* Los Angeles, CA: Western Psychological Services Inc.

Pfeiffer, B. A., Koenig, K., Kinnealey, M., Sheppard, M., & Henderson, L. (2011). Effectiveness of sensory integration interventions in children with autism spectrum disorders: A pilot study. *American Journal of Occupational Therapy, 65,* 76-85.

Reichow, B., Doehring, P., Cicchetti, D. V., & Volkmar, F. R. (2011). *Evidence-based practices and treatments for children with autism.* New York, NY: Springer.

Reisman, J., & Hanschu, B. (1992). *Sensory integration – Revised for individuals with developmental disabilities: User's guide.* Hugo, MN: PDP Press.

Reynolds, S., & Lane, S. J. (2008). Diagnostic validity of sensory overresponsivity: A review of the literature and case reports. *Journal of Autism and Developmental Disorders, 38,* 516-529.

Rosenhall, U., Nordin, V., Brantberg, K., & Gillberg, C. (2003). Autism and auditory brain stem responses. *Ear and Hearing, 24,* 206-214.

Schaaf, R. C., Benevides, T. W., Leiby, B. E., & Sendecki, J. A. (2013). Autonomic dysregulation during sensory stimulation in children with autism spectrum disorder. *Journal of Autism and Developmental Disorders.* doi:10.1007/s10803-013-1924-6

Schertz, H. H., Baker, C., Hurwitz, S., & Benner, L. (2011). Principles of early intervention reflected in toddler research in autism spectrum disorders. *Topics in Early Childhood Special Education, 31*(1), 4-21.

Shochat, T., Tzischinsky, O., & Engel-Yeger, B. (2009). Sensory hypersensitivity as a contributing factor in the relation between sleep and behavioral disorders in normal school children. *Behavioral Sleep Medicine, 7,* 53-62.

Shore, S. (2003). *Beyond the wall: Personal experiences with autism and Asperger Syndrome* (2nd ed.). Shawnee Mission, KS: AAPC Publishing.

Smith, S. A., Press, B., Koenig, K. P., & Kinnealey, M. (2005). Effects of sensory integration intervention on self-stimulating and self-injurious behaviors. *American Journal of Occupational Therapy, 59,* 418-425.

Smith, S. M., Myles, B. S., Aspy, R., Grossman, B. G., & Henry, S. (2010). Sustainable change in quality of life for individuals with ASD: Using a comprehensive planning process. *Focus on Exceptional Children, 43*(3), 1-24.

Takarae, Y., Luna, B., Minshew, N. J., & Sweeneys, J. A. (2008). Patterns of visual sensory and sensomotor abnormalities in autism vary in relation to history of early language delay. *Journal of the International Neuropsychological Society, 14*(6), 980-989. doi:10.1017/S1355617708081277

Tavassoli, T., Latham, K., Bach, M., Dakin, S. C., & Baron-Cohen, S. (2011). Psychophysical measures of visual acuity in autism spectrum conditions. *Vision Research, 51,* 1778-1780.

Texas Statewide Leadership for Autism Training. (2011). *Final report.* Retrieved from http://www.txautism.net

Tomchek, S. D., & Dunn, W. (2007). Sensory processing in children with and without autism: A comparative study using the short sensory profile. *The American Journal of Occupational Therapy, 61,* 190-200.

Van Steensel, F. J. A., Bögels, S. M., & Perrin, S. (2011). Anxiety disorders in children and adolescents with autism spectrum disorders: A meta-analysis. *Clinical Child and Family Psychology Review, 14,* 302-317.

Veenendall, J. (2009). *Why does Izzy cover her ears? Dealing with sensory overload.* Shawnee Mission, KS: AAPC Publishing.

Veenendall, J. (2010). *Arnie and his school tools: Simple sensory solutions that build success.* Shawnee Mission, KS: AAPC Publishing.

Vernazza-Martin, S., Martin, N., Vernazza, A., Lepellec-Muller, A., Rufo, M., Massion, J., & Assaiante, C. (2005). Goal-directed locomotion and balance control in autistic children. *Journal of Autism and Developmental Disorders, 35,* 91-102.

Weimer, A. K., Schatz, A. M., Lincoln, A., Ballantyne, A. O., & Trauner, D. A. (2001). "Motor" impairment in Asperger syndrome: Evidence for a deficit in proprioception. *Developmental and Behavioral Pediatrics, 22,* 92-101.

Williams, M. W., & Shellenberger, S. (1996). *How does your engine run? A leader's guide to the Alert Program for Self-Regulation.* Albuquerque, NM: TherapyWorks.

Wing, L. (1981). Asperger Syndrome: A clinical account. *Psychological Medicine, 11,* 115-129.

Witt, J. C., VanDerHeyden, A. M., & Gilbertson, D. (2004). Troubleshooting behavioral interventions: A systematic process for finding and eliminating problems. *School Psychology Review, 33*(3), 363-383.

Woods, J. J., & Brown, J. A. (2011). Integrating family capacity-building and child outcomes to support communication development in young children with autism spectrum disorders. *Topics in Language Disorders, 31*(3), 235-246.

Yack, E., Sutton, S., & Aquilla, P. (2003). *Building bridges through sensory integration: Therapy for children with autism and other pervasive developmental disorders.* Arlington, TX: Future Horizons.

RESOURCES
Toys and Materials

Abledata
8455 Colesville Rd., Suite 935
Silver Spring, MD 20910-3319
800-227-0216
abledata.com

Listings of over 19,000 products for individuals with disabilities, including information about toys for children with special needs.

Achievement Products, Inc.
P.O. Box 9033
Canton, OH 44711
800-373-4699
AchievementProductsInc.com

Catalog of special education and rehabilitation equipment for children with special needs from birth to 18.

Autism Resource Network, Inc.
5123 Westmill Rd.
Minnetonka, MN 55345
612-988-0088
autismbooks.com

Books and materials with emphasis on AS and autism.

Childgarden
P.O. Box 15023
St. Louis, MO 63110
800-726-4769
childgarden.com

Pillows, cuddle-ups (large-sized pillows that look like animals/bugs).

Childswork/Childsplay Center
P.O. Box 61586
King of Prussia, PA 19406
800-962-1141
childswork.com

A catalog designed to address the mental health needs of children and families through play with books, board games, puppets, posters, videos, dolls, and doll houses.

Communication Skill Builders, Inc.
555 Academic Ct.
San Antonio, TX 78204-2498
800-211-8378
hbtpc.com

Therapy resources and books with an emphasis on communication.

Community Playthings
P.O. Box 901
Rifton, NY 12471-0901
800-777-4244
communityproducts.com

Although not specially designed for children with special needs, many of the products may be of interest.

Constructive Playthings
1227 East 119th St.
Grandview, MO 64030-1117
816-761-5900
constructiveplaythings.com

Although not specially designed for children with special needs, many of the products may be of interest.

Discount School Supply
 PO Box 6013
Carol Stream, IL 60197-6013
800-627-2829
discountschoolsupply.com

Art materials, containers, Velcro, and other useful items.

Don Johnston, Inc.
P.O. Box 639
1000 N. Rand Rd., Bldg. 115
Wauconda, IL 60084
800-999-4660
donjohnston.com

Computer software, hardware, and switches.

Fun and Function
POB 11, Merion Station, PA 19066
funandfunction.com

Toys, equipment and supplies to support sensory regulation, motor skill development and play skills.

Lakeshore Learning Materials
2965 E. Dominques
Carson, CA 90749
800-421-5354
lakeshorelearning.com

Educational products, adaptive equipment, and outdoor play equipment.

Mayer-Johnson Co.
P.O. Box 1579
Solana Beach, CA 92075-7579
800-588-4548
mayer-johnson.com

Communication system software (great for PECS systems), including books, materials and resources.

National Autism Resources
6240 Goodyear Rd.
Benicia, CA 94510
nationalautismresources.com

Toys, products, books, equipment for individuals with ASD.

One Step Ahead
P.O. Box 517
Lake Bluff, IL 60044
800-274-8440
onestepahead.com

Although not specifically designed
for children with special needs, many
of the products may be of interest
(for children from newborn through
kindergarten age).

Oriental Trading Company, Inc.
P.O. Box 2308
Omaha, NE 68103-2308
800-228-2269
orientaltrading.com

Inexpensive bulk items great for
reinforcers, fidgets, and other sensory
needs.

PDP Products
P.O. Box 2009
Stillwater, MN 55082
651-439-8865
pdppro.com

Books, sensory materials for fidgets,
and fun toys.

Perfectly Safe
The Catalog Designed for
Parents Who Care
7245 Whipple Ave. NW
North Canton, OH 44270
800-837-KIDS (5437)
kidsstuff.com

Although not specifically designed
for children with special needs, many
of the products may be of interest; all
are designed to ensure child safety.

Play with a Purpose
220 24th Ave. NW
P.O. Box 998
Owatonna, MN 55060-0998
800-533-0446
gophersport.com

Toys, materials, and games that emphasize physical development, gross-
and fine-motor skills, and play.

Pocket Full of Therapy
P.O. Box 174
Morganville, NJ 07751
pfot.com

Toys, equipment and supplies that
support sensory regulation and motor skill development.

Pro-Ed
8700 Shoal Creek Blvd.
Austin, TX 78757-6897
800-897-3202
proedinc.com

Tests, reference books, journals, etc.,
used in educational settings.

**Raymond Geddes and
Company, Inc.**
P.O. Box 24829
Baltimore, MD 21220-0829
800-533-6273
raymondgeddes.com

Inexpensive items, stickers, pencil
toppers, and fidgets for sensory
needs.

Rifton Equipment
P.O. Box 901, Route 213
Rifton, NY 12471
800-777-4244
communityproducts.com

Specialized equipment for children
with disabilities.

Sammons Preston
An AbilityOne Company
P.O. Box 5071
Bolingbrook, IL 60440-5071
800-323-5547
sammonspreston.com

Positioning, seating, mobility, and
recreational and adaptive devices for
individuals with special needs.

SmileMakers
P.O. Box 2543
Spartanburg, SC 29304
800-825-8085
smilemakers.com

Fidgets, stickers, small sensory items,
and reinforcers at inexpensive
prices.

Southpaw Enterprises, Inc.
P.O. Box 1047
Dayton, OH 45401-1047
800-228-1698
southpawenterprises.com

Catalog of sensory integration and
developmental therapy products.

Sportime/Abilitiations
One Sportime Way
Atlanta, GA 30340
800-850-8602
abilitations.com

Recreation and exercise products.

Therapro
225 Arlington St.
Framingham, MA 01702-8723
800-257-5376
theraproducts.com

Catalog of resources/materials for
parents, educators, and therapists.

Therapy Shoppe
P.O. Box 8875
Grand Rapids, MI 49518
therapyshoppe.com

Specialize in sensory integration
products, special needs toys, oral motor tools, and occupational therapy
supplies.

RESOURCES
Organizations

American Occupational Therapy Association, Inc.
4720 Montgomery Lane
Bethesda, MD 20824-1220
301-652-AOTA or
1-800-668-8255
aota.org

American Physical Therapy Association
1111 North Fairfax St.
Alexandria, VA 22314-1488
703-684-2782
apta.org

American Speech-LanguageHearing Association
10801 Rockville Pike
Rockville, MD 20852
301-897-5700 or 800-638-TALK
asha.org

Autism Society
4350 East-West Highway, Suite 350
Bethesda, MD 20814800-3AUTISM
autism-society.org

Autism Speaks
1 East 33rd Street 4th Floor New York, NY 10016
autismspeaks.org

Council for Exceptional Children (CEC)
1920 Association Dr.
Reston, VA 22091
703-620-3660
cecsped.org

Geneva Center for Autism
250 Davisville Ave., Suite 200
Toronto, Ontario
Canada M4S 1H2
416-322-7877
autism.net

OASIS @ MAAP
aspergersyndrome.org

Sensory Processing Disorder Foundation
5420 S. Quebec Street, Suite 135
Greenwood Village, CO 80111
spdfoundation.net
sinetwork.org

TherapyWorks Inc.
4901 Butte Pl., NW
Albuquerque, NM 87120
505-897-3478
alertprogram.com

Western Psychological Services
Sensory Integration Training
12031 Wilshire Blvd.
Los Angeles, CA 90025-1251
800-648-8857
wpspublish.com

Many of the national organizations have state chapters. Each national organization can give you information about your state's chapter.

RELATED BOOKS FROM AAPC

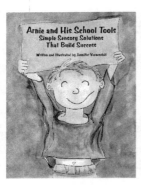

Arnie and His School Tools

Simple Sensory Solutions That Build Success

written and illustrated by Jennifer Veenendall

This illustrated children's book centers around an exuberant boy who had difficulty paying attention in class and doing his schoolwork until he was equipped with tools that helped accommodate his sensory needs. The book uses simple language to describe some of the sensory tools and strategies Arnie uses at school and at home to help him achieve a more optimal level of alertness and performance. Additional resources are provided at the end of the book, including definitions of sensory processing and sensory modulation disorder, suggested discussion questions and lists of related books and websites.

ISBN 9781934575154 | Code 9002 | Price: $18.95

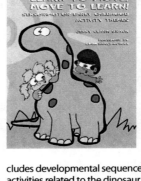

Learn to Move, Move to Learn!

Sensorimotor Early Childhood Activity Themes

by Jenny Clark Brack, OTR/L, BCP AOTA Board Certification in Pediatrics

Learn to Move, Move to Learn features an evidence-based sensory integration program that includes developmental sequences consisting of seven activities related to the dinosaur theme. Suggestions for adaptation and modification for individual students are included, along with instructions for how to develop additional lessons. The companion DVD, *Learn to Move, Move to Learn: Dinosaurs*, gives a first-hand view of real children engaged in a theme-based sensorimotor lesson and thus sparks ideas for other similar activities.

ISBN 9781931282635 | Code 9943 | Price: $34.95

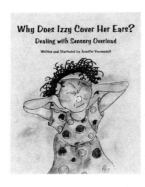

Why Does Izzy Cover Her Ears?

Dealing With Sensory Overload

written and illustrated by Jennifer Veenendall

Meet Izzy, a feisty first grader, whose behavior is often misunderstood as she tries to cope with sensory overload in her new surroundings. This brightly illustrated book creates an environment that is accepting of students with sensory modulation difficulties, including many on the autism spectrum. It's a great resource for occupational therapists, teachers, and parents to share with children. Resources for adults at the end of the book include definitions of sensory processing and sensory modulation disorder, suggested discussion questions and lists of related books and web sites.

ISBN 9781934575468 | Code 9037 | Price: $18.95

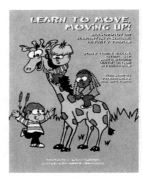

Learn to Move, Moving Up!

Sensorimotor Elementary-School Activity Themes

by Jenny Clark Brack, OTR/L, BCP AOTA Board Certification in Pediatrics

Using the same easy-to-use format as her first book, *Learn to Move, Move to Learn*, Jenny Clark now brings a series of sensory-based activities for older school-aged children. These literacy-rich lesson plans include specially designed curriculum suggestions and underscore how activities can be adapted to meet state and other standards. The book also contains a thorough, up-to-date discussion of sensory integration and sensory processing disorders; assessment and evaluation considerations, including a reproducible Teacher Observation Checklist; evidence-based best-practice strategies; how to integrate lessons into elementary school environments; as well as learning enrichment suggestions.

ISBN 9781934575383 | Code 9024 | Price: $34.95

Order online at www.aapcpublishing.net

RELATED BOOKS FROM AAPC

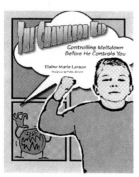

The Chameleon Kid

Controlling Meltdown Before He Controls You

by Elaine M. Larson

For a child with ASD, meltdowns are often frequent, explosive, long-lasting events. *The Chameleon Kid* encourages children to control the Meltdown lurking inside them by evoking the adaptable abilities of the chameleon. Colorful illustrations and short verses present the various reactions that "the bad guy" Meltdown can cause, followed by advice for how the Chameleon Kid can adapt his emotions and attitudes to prevent Meltdown from taking over. In the process, readers learn various methods of self-regulating their emotion.

ISBN 9781934575222 | Code 9010 | Price: $18.95

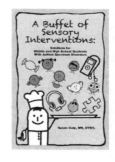

A Buffet of Sensory Interventions:

Solutions for Middle and High School Students With Autism Spectrum Disorders

by Susan Culp, MS, OTR/L

A Buffet of Sensory Interventions focuses on middle and high school students whose sensory needs are often overlooked. The book emphasizes the importance of fostering independence, self-advocacy and self-regulation as a way for teens with autism spectrum disorders to take ownership of their needs as they transition into adulthood. Using simple terminology and lots of illustrations, it explains sensory integration basics, and helps develop daily interventions through assessment of sensory needs.

ISBN 9781934575833 | Code 9058 | Price: $19.95

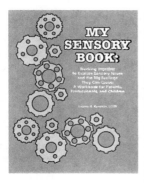

My Sensory Book:

Working Together to Explore Sensory Issues and the Big Feelings They Can Cause: A Workbook for Parents, Professionals, and Children

by Lauren H. Kerstein, LCSW

My Sensory Book enables children to develop a better understanding of their sensory systems by helping their parents and teachers create an individualized sensory profile. Through numerous strategies broken down by the different sensory systems – tactile, vestibular, proprioception, visual, auditory, gustatory and olfactory – children can learn to cope more effectively with the world around them. This is a practical tool for both home and school.

ISBN 9781934575215 | Code 9006 | Price: $21.95

Order online at www.aapcpublishing.net

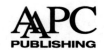

P.O. Box 23173
Shawnee Mission, Kansas 66283-0173
www.aapcpublishing.net

CPSIA information can be obtained at www.ICGtesting.com
Printed in the USA
LVOW12s0332250714

395682LV00006B/9/P